# Introduction

Teresa Thompson

*Department of Communication*
*University of Dayton*

The origin of this special issue of *Health Communication* (*HC*) was a panel at the annual conference of the International Communication Association several years ago. The panel, planned by Kelly McNeilis, focused on the description of provider–patient interaction coding systems. Several of the authors of essays in this issue participated in that panel. I was the respondent. Both the audience members and I were struck by the different aspects of provider–patient interaction assessed by the various coding systems described on the panel. Someone suggested that it would be interesting to have the same data set coded by the different coding systems. It would allow a more accurate assessment of the various conclusions that came out of the application of different coding schema. Thus, this issue was begun.

We originally hoped to put together a book in which the authors would be able to thoroughly and completely describe their coding systems as well as report the results of their analyses of the same data set. This would have been advantageous, in that it would have provided a forum in which other researchers could find complete details of most of the key coding systems available all in one place instead of having to hunt up dozens of sources. We feared that there would not be a large enough market for such a volume, however, and decided to go with a special issue of *HC* instead.

The videotaped data analyzed by the research reports found herein were made available to us by Marlene von Friederichs-Fitzwater. Our thanks go to her. The tapes were interactions of residents, attending physicians, and patients and included analysis of a number of health problems. There were 10 interactions, 8 of which involved both an attending physician and a resident. The patients, approximately half men and half women, were ethnically diverse, including Whites, African Americans, and Hispanics. All patients were lower income. Four of the

Requests for reprints should be sent to Teresa Thompson, Department of Communication, University of Dayton, Dayton, OH 45469–1410. E-mail: thompson@udayton.edu

physicians were women. All the interactions were first time visits to a family practice clinic at an urban teaching medical center. The interactions ranged in length from 19 to 45 min with an average of 32 min. They included such health issues as the management of chronic disease, multiple injuries, and an initial prenatal visit.

As is the case with much real-world data, parts of the videotapes were difficult to understand. Two of the interactions were not analyzed by some of the research teams because too much was inaudible.

Some of the coding systems described in this issue involve coding directly from video, others from audio, and others from transcripts. The researchers who coded from transcripts split up the videotapes and shared their transcriptions with each other. I thank Bill Stiles for coordinating this.

This issue does not, of course, include all possible provider–patient interaction coding schemes. In particular, we had hoped to include Ron Adelman and Michelle Greene's coding system (e.g., see Charon, Greene, & Adelman, 1994) and were unable to do so. Their coding system requires the coding of an entire interaction, and some parts of some of the coded interactions were missing due to privacy concerns or inaudibility. We had also at one point hoped to relate the interaction data to medical outcome data, but some of the authors argued against doing so (e.g., see Stiles, 1989). We also did not have a data set available (for confidentiality and informed consent reasons) that would have allowed us to do so. Data sets collected for one purpose cannot typically be made available to other researchers. We were lucky that von Friederichs-Fitzwater's data were available.

As you read the essays, you will find that the coding systems utilized focus in some ways on very different aspects of interaction. The Roter and Larson article, using the Roter Interaction Analysis System (RIAS), focuses on the differences between the residents' and attendings' communication because the researchers were initially intrigued by the differences they noticed. The researchers describe both the frequencies of the various categories of interaction and the relations among those categories. The RIAS, based on a social exchange perspective, is probably the most frequently utilized coding scheme of all those described in this issue.

The Meredith, Stewart, and Belle Brown article utilizes a patient-centered communication coding scheme. The theoretical orientation underlying this schema leads to a focus on just certain types of behaviors—those that notably are or are not patient centered. These categories tend to be broader than those found in some of the other systems, and lead to a noticeably more evaluative analysis of the degree of patient centeredness of a particular interaction.

Bill Stiles and two of his graduate students, Ayesha Shaikh and Lynne Knobloch, report an analysis of the interactions using his Verbal Response Mode (VRM) coding system. The VRM, which has been applied to a variety of other interactional contexts as well as the medical interaction, focuses on roles as defined by communication and emphasizes the status and relational aspects of those roles. There are three key bipolar role dimensions assessed by the VRM. This research team examined differences among the medical history, physical examination, and concluding segments of the interactions.

Perhaps the most extensive of the coding systems in the present issue is described by Kelly McNeilis. Based on the Cegala and Waldron (1992) model of communicative competence, the McNeilis Coordination and Competence System (CACS) focuses on both the alignment and the function of messages. This article utilizes lag sequential analysis to assess patterns of interaction; the results demonstrate the kinds of responses likely to be elicited by particular message types. McNeilis thus provides a more directly dyadic, interactional perspective than do most coding schemes. Additionally, her schema is based on initial research demonstrating those behaviors that are judged as more versus less competent in the medical context.

The only coding system to report both quantitative and qualitative assessments is found in the article by Rick Street and Bradford Millay. Street and Millay focus particularly on patient participation in the medical encounter. They code four types of patient participation and two types of physician patient-centered responses to examine interrelationships amongst them. The coding system explicitly relies on nonverbals to determine the categorizations of verbal statements, although this reliance is implicit in many of the other coding systems. Street and Millay note that patients' acts of participation appear to encourage the physicians to be more patient-centered, and that encouraging patient participation does not require longer interactions.

The most unusual coding, Relational Control Coding, is reported in the article by Marlene von Friederichs-Fitzwater and John Gilgun. Relational coding was not originally developed for the medical context, but has now been applied to it by a number of researchers. Rather than focusing on message content, relational coding looks at interactional control as it is manifested by each communicative act. It then looks at patterns of control determined by interacts. This perspective, like several others, relates to a patient-centered view of medical interaction. The results of this analysis, however, demonstrate a more doctor- or disease-centered pattern in the coded interactions.

The reader will note different interpretations of the interactions and different conclusions arising from the applications of the various coding schemes. Raijv Rimal comments on some of these differences in his response to the research reports, as well as suggesting some new directions for the study of provider–patient interaction. Rimal refers to the studies in alphabetical order by first author, so I have arranged them in that order within this issue as well.

Rimal's response is followed by one by Richard Frankel, who was asked to respond to this issue because his perspective and work on provider–patient interaction is rather different than those found in most of the quantitative analyses reported herein. Frankel's response begins with a historical overview of research on provider–patient interaction and then moves to a discussion of the various analyses in this issue. He discusses how the nature of the various coding schemes leads the researchers to notice different aspects of the interactions and ignore other aspects. He places the findings in the broader context of the study of provider–patient interaction. He also cómments on some practical and methodological conclusions that arise from the comparisons of the various perspectives.

The various coding schemes described herein definitely offer different foci and emphases and are appropriate for slightly different purposes. Our goal in this issue is to provide a resource that will make it easier for future researchers to select a coding scheme that is most appropriate for the purpose of a particular research project. It is hoped, then, that this issue will help illuminate the process of studying health care provider–patient interaction and will facilitate decision making for future researchers. Enjoy your reading!

## REFERENCES

Cegala, D., & Waldron, V. (1992). A study of the relationship between communicative performance and conversation participants' thoughts. *Communication Studies, 43,* 105–123.

Charon, R., Greene, M. G., & Adelman, R. D. (1994). Multi-dimensional interaction analysis: A collaborative approach to the study of medical discourse. *Social Science and Medicine, 39,* 955–965.

Stiles, W. B. (1989). Evaluating medical interview process components: Null correlations with outcomes may be misleading. *Medical Care, 27,* 212–220.

# Analyzing Communication Competence in Medical Consultations

## Kelly S. McNeilis

*Department of Communication and Mass Media*
*Southwest Missouri State University*

One approach to understanding and illuminating communicative processes in the medical consultation is to directly analyze discourse features within the interview. The model advanced here examines sequential properties of talk in the medical consultation to identify competent patterns of communication. Competence is observed in terms of participants' abilities to align their utterances in the service of meeting both self and other goals. In this article, the Coordination and Competence System (CACS; Gillotti, Thompson, & McNeilis, in press) and its conceptual foundation of communication competence will be explained along with results of its application to sample interactions. Finally, conclusions about communication competence in medical consultations will be discussed in terms of important results and directions for future research.

## CONCEPTUAL FRAMEWORK FOR CODING SYSTEM

One of the more enduring conceptual and theoretical traditions in speech communication has been the study of communication competence. Cegala and Waldron's (1992) context-bound model of communication competence serves as the conceptual framework for this research. In this model, emphasis is placed on participants' communicative behavior and on how people align their utterances in coordinating their goals. The notion of alignment implies that competent communicators interpret and produce messages that facilitate individual and mutual goals. Such alignment entails participants' attention to the intent and meaning of each other's mes-

Requests for reprints should be sent to Kelly S. McNeilis, Department of Communication, Southwest Missouri State University, 901 South National Avenue, Springfield, MO 65804. E-mail: ksm911f@ smsu.edu

sages, and construction of subsequent utterances to meet the concerns of the interlocutor. Applied to physician–patient interactions, theorizing about competence involves identifying competent interactions and then using those observations and patterns to assist in providing communication skills training to patients and physicians, among other outcomes. In doing so, we describe how coordination is accomplished, at what level, and also the function that utterance is serving (task being accomplished) in the medical interview. Generally, medical interactions involve the tasks of information exchange and socioemotional concern.

The coding scheme reported here is a modified version of the original (McNeilis, 1995). The CACS was developed to identify communication competence and centers on three primary criteria—message content, alignment, and function. A secondary criterion of the coding scheme involves two aspects of interaction management—acknowledgment tokens and interruptions. Due to space limitations only alignment and function are explained here.

Although minimum requirements of alignment occur at the global level, additional requirements are found at lower levels of discourse. Because alignment is concerned with the extent to which a subsequent utterance fits with a prior utterance, it also may be assessed on local grounds. For example, participants may both address a common global content theme (e.g., the weather), but their utterances may be misaligned in terms of function (e.g., a question is not adequately answered or is ignored entirely). Thus, what may be coherent, aligned discourse at one level may be incoherent and disjointed at another level. The assumption here is that successful coordination of goals requires alignment on multiple levels of discourse.

As indicated already, one component of the coding system is concerned with interaction management (Wiemann, 1977), and involves matters of timing, turn taking, and regulation through continuous feedback. In particular, acknowledgment tokens and interruptions are coded, although interruptions are not the focus of this analysis. A second way in which utterance fit is defined is in terms of local topic synchronization or uptake. Here, utterances are coded for such matters as topic change and issue versus event extensions. The major objective of such assessment is to index the extent to which participants fashion their utterances to address central, peripheral, or different substantive matters of the interlocutor's previous utterance. For more information on the development of this level, consult Gillotti et al. (in press).

Finally, the third way in which utterance alignment is defined is with respect to how utterances mesh functionally. For example, in most instances participants expect an answer to follow a question. Such expectation for functional fit contributes to participants' experience and assessment of conversational coherence. In the current coding system, there are 25 functional categories, many of which reflect the basic goals of information exchange and relational development in the medical consultation.

## CODING PROCEDURES AND APPLICATION

The coding system used in this analysis is a simplified version of the original (McNeilis, 1995). For this project only two levels were coded—alignment and function of utterances. Revisions have been made including subsuming some categories, and elaborating on others. For instance, previous codes including reinforcement, naming, and legitimizing affect were subsumed into the relational category. Some codes were eliminated and subsumed into others to use a sequential analysis program most effectively.

The coding unit is the utterance. The definition of an *utterance* used here is a word or series of words spoken by an individual constituting a thought or partial thought and that may or may not be interrupted by or overlapped with other talk by the partner. If there is an overlap, the first unit ends there and the next unit begins with the overlapped talk. Multiple utterances can occur within one speaking turn. The obtained reliability for unitizing using Holsti's (1969) method is .96 as reported by Gillotti et al. (in press).

After unitizing is completed, the coding can begin. First, alignment is coded for each utterance. Alignment has five primary codes. These identify the extent to which an utterance is responsive to the previous utterance. The extent to which doctors and patients align their utterances by picking up (uptaking) on a topic or theme of importance to the interlocutor is considered important to the ultimate coordination of goals. Thus, topic continuation is a relevant feature of coordination. *Issue* and *event* topic extensions (Tracy, 1982) denote coordination because they have been shown to be related to perceptions of competence. In addition, *continuers,* brief utterances of one or two words inviting more talk on the topic, are relevant to alignment. Additionally, when a participant changes the theme of the discussion altogether, we have included topic changes as another feature. A *topic change* occurs when the new topic introduced is substantively different from the topic of the previous utterance. The final feature included in alignment is *pop extensions,* which occur when a participant refers back to a topic that has been already discussed.

Once alignment level is identified for each unit, a function code is assigned to each unit. Function identifies the main purpose being served by a turn. In other words, what a turn "does" or accomplishes is considered a function. Some of the function codes in the scheme are specific to the medical interview setting, whereas others are applicable to any conversation. The function categories are broadly represented within five general categories that are related to tasks in the medical interview: Information seeking, information giving, information verifying, socioemotional, and other. Codes 1 and 2 are intended to assess aspects of information seeking including questions and embedded questions (seeking information but embedded within a declarative statement). Codes 3 through 9 assess information-giving strategies including solicited answers, elaborations, unsolicited information, expansions, assertions, justifications, and explanations. Codes 10 through 13 assess information-verifying strategies and include conditionally relevant questions, formulations, restatements, and foreshadowing (formerly bracketing; McNeilis, 1995). Codes 14 through 19 assess the extent to which an utterance serves a socioemotional function. These statements serve to reinforce a relational perception, to change it, or to modify it, and generally are referred to as relationship-building attempts by the participants. Specifically these are relational statements, apologies, hedging, small talk, acknowledgment tokens, and humor. Acknowledgment tokens are a conversational management strategy that signify simple recognition or confirmation of the partner's previous turn and receipt of information (e.g., P: "Yeah, and I'd like you to check on that mole that I told you popped up last month." D: "Okay, let's move onto the examination then ... "). Finally, additional function Codes 20 to 25 identify instances of agreement, disagreement, corrections, directives, compliance, and incomplete units.

Independent coders not associated with the project have established coding reliability of the system. Some coders were a part of the original research report of the coding scheme, whereas others were a group of undergraduate students who worked on a class project at another university (Gillotti et al., in press). Holsti's (1969) method of agreement was used to determine reliability scores on each of the codes. Cohen's kappa is also an acceptable and more conservative method. Reliability scores have been recorded as ranging from .76 to .85 for alignment, .70 to .87 for function, and .68 to .72 for acknowledgment tokens (this unique code indicates alignment and has no function code assigned).

## RESULTS

Two sets of results are reported in this section. First, frequency data for the individual categories are presented in Tables 1 and 2. Second, the more unique sequential analysis results are reported in detail.

Because of space limitations, frequency results presented in Tables 1 and 2 are not discussed explicitly. For these data, a total of 3,922 units were coded from the 10 doctor–patient interviews provided. Of this total, 55% (2,148) of the units were contributed by the doctors, and the remaining 45% (1,774) of the units were provided by the patients in this sample.

A few of the results are noted as a precursor to interpreting the sequential analysis results. First, questions and answers are unequally distributed between doctors and patients. Second, topic control was accomplished primarily by the physicians. Patients in this sample asked relatively few direct questions and the doctors provided few answers and elaborations in response. Finally, there is a distinct lack of relationship-building statements in these interviews. These are key to understanding the patterns of interaction noted in the next section.

TABLE 1
Frequencies and Proportions of Alignment Codes by Role

| Alignments Codes | Doctors | | Patients | | Total |
|---|---|---|---|---|---|
| | f | Proportion | f | Proportion | |
| Issue extensions | 902 | .502 | 1,319 | .841 | 2,221 |
| Event extensions | 403 | .224 | 137 | .087 | 540 |
| Topic changes | 229 | .127 | 14 | .008 | 243 |
| Pop extensions | 70 | .039 | 10 | .007 | 80 |
| Continuers | 192 | .106 | 87 | .005 | 279 |
| Totals[a] | 1,796 | | 1,567 | | 3,363 |

*Note.* All results reported in this table indicate raw frequencies of each category regardless of function code.

[a]These totals do not add up to unit totals for function categories in Table 2. Laughter, acknowledgment tokens, incompletes, humor, and hedges do not have alignment codes assigned.

## Sequential Analysis Findings

Interactive data require sequential analyses programs to identify patterns. Lags (given one behavior what behavior occurs next) are computed and can be checked for the statistical significance that one pattern of codes occurred with a greater proportion than another. For these data, the general sequential querier (GSEQ; Bakeman & Quera, 1995) was used on all codes. Commands are given to identify frequencies and significance of specific codes and what follows immediately after (Lag 1). Two steps after one code would be identified as Lag 2.

To identify competent patterns, initial criteria for competent exchanges were identified by McNeilis and Cegala (1997) and further elaborated by Cegala, Coleman, and Turner (1998). The criteria developed generally focused on information exchange and relational competence including how patient-initiated topics are followed up on, how detailed doctors' explanations are, and how the participants show positivity to one another. First, alignment moves are reported and then second function categories and their sequences are noted for competent and less competent patterns.

*Alignment.* In identifying competent aligning moves, notable results for who initiated topic changes and topic follow-up emerged. In these data, 94% of the topic changes ($n = 229$) were made by physicians. Ideally there would be equal opportunity for patients and physicians to choose from all alignment moves, specifically in regard to changing topics. In an effort to understand what may prompt a doctor to change the subject, analyses were conducted on what comes before topic changes. Results of sequential analysis showed no significant pattern of what preceded topic changes. The only result of note was a pattern whereby doctors changed the topic

TABLE 2
Frequencies and Proportions of Language Categories by Role

| Function Categories | | Doctor | | Patient | | |
|---|---|---|---|---|---|---|
| | | f | Proportion | f | Proportion | Totals |
| Information seeking | Questions | 742 | .38 | 35 | .02 | 777 |
| | Embedded questions | 4 | .002 | 26 | .01 | 30 |
| Information giving | Solicited answers | 24 | .01 | 632 | .37 | 656 |
| | Elaborations | 2 | .001 | 72 | .04 | 74 |
| | Unsolicited information | 6 | .003 | 68 | .04 | 74 |
| | Expansions | 67 | .03 | 311 | .18 | 378 |
| | Assertions | 92 | .04 | 91 | .05 | 183 |
| | Justification | 56 | .02 | 4 | .002 | 60 |
| | Explanations | 115 | .06 | 2 | .001 | 117 |
| Information verifying | Conditionally relevant questions | 24 | .01 | 14 | .007 | 38 |
| | Formulations | 77 | .04 | 2 | .001 | 79 |
| | Restatements | 89 | .05 | 13 | .007 | 102 |
| | Foreshadowing | 50 | .02 | 0 | | 50 |
| Socioemotional | Relational statements | 108 | .05 | 22 | .01 | 130 |
| | Apologies | 6 | .002 | 3 | .001 | 9 |
| | Hedges | 1 | .000 | 2 | .001 | 3 |
| | Small talk | 34 | .01 | 32 | .02 | 66 |
| | Laughter | 6 | .002 | 16 | .009 | 22 |
| | Humor | 7 | .003 | 3 | .001 | 10 |
| | Acknowledgment tokens (freestanding) | 288 | .15 | 119 | .07 | 407 |
| Other | Corrections | 7 | .002 | 8 | .004 | 15 |
| | Disagreements | 1 | .000 | 2 | .001 | 3 |
| | Agreements | 18 | .008 | 123 | .07 | 141 |
| | Directives | 79 | .04 | 0 | | 79 |
| | Compliance | 2 | .001 | 19 | .01 | 21 |
| | 1st utterance question | 0 | | 1 | .000 | 1 |
| | 1st utterance relational | 0 | | 1 | .000 | 1 |
| | Incompletes | 51 | .03 | 66 | .04 | 117 |
| | Total units | 1,956 | | 1,687 | | 3,643 |

*Note.*   All results reported in this table indicate raw frequencies of each function category across all alignment codes. Proportions have been rounded.

with a question (*n* = 26) after patients' acknowledgment tokens. Perhaps doctors see these tokens as openings to move forward and an indication of patient understanding. This could be a dangerous assumption given that acknowledgment tokens are just that, tokens that "I've heard you," but not necessarily that "I understand." This pattern of frequent topic shifts by physicians may not allow patients adequate time to comprehend or to process information shared by the physician. No results of note could be found in looking at what proceeded or followed patient topic changes. This is due in part to relatively few patient topic changes (*n* = 14). We discuss implications for health communication research in this area in the conclusions.

*Function.*     This section describes patterns of functional categories and their frequency. These results revolve around three groups of tasks accomplished in the medical interview: information exchange, information verifying, and socioemotional tasks. Due to space limitations, selected findings are reported.

Information exchange competence involves the extent to which doctors and patients provide information to and seek it out from one another relatively equally. This competence criteria is partially evident in these data. Patients primarily provided issue-relevant information and physicians primarily sought information. In spite of that finding, Cegala and his colleagues (Cegala et al., 1998; Cegala, McGee, & McNeilis, 1996; Cegala, McNeilis, McGee, & Jonas, 1995) have reported that information seeking, giving, and verifying ranked highest on both doctors and patients' thoughts during the medical interview. In addition, they reported that these issues are relevant to communication competence. As such, information seeking on the part of patients and follow-up on patient-initiated topics seem to be additional components of competence related to information exchange (McNeilis, 1995).

To identify the sequences of competent and less competent information exchange, the reader must attend to the following question: What are the participants doing in their talk to be responsive to each other's goals? To answer this question, specific sequences of information seeking, giving, and the like are explored to identify how information exchange goals are accomplished more or less competently.

First, we look at information seeking. Not surprisingly doctors' attempts at requesting information were met with solicited answers by patients most frequently (see Table 3). Doctors and patients in this sample were extremely adept in their respective roles. One of the more glaring issues regarding information-seeking goals involved attempts by patients to ask questions and the responses offered by physicians. In general, patients asked few questions of their physicians very competently, as evidenced in proportionally few direct and embedded questions posed (see Table 2). Embedded questions, although at least exhibiting a moderate amount of competence, still may not prompt the kind of information desired. As such, what happens after embedded questions was explored. A competent response to embedded questions would be to provide a direct answer, explanation, or

TABLE 3
Selected Information Exchange Sequences Pooled Over 10 Dyads

| | "Y" Followed | | | | | |
| | Responses to Questions—Information Giving | | | | | |
| Given "X" | E Solicited | I Solicited | E Elab. | I Elab. | E Unsolicited | I Unsolicited |
|---|---|---|---|---|---|---|
| Event questions | 4 | 224 | 3 | 24 | 2 | 1 |
| Issue questions | 2 | 282 | 1 | 23 | 3 | 1 |

| | Responses to Answers—Information Verifying and Follow-up | | | |
| | I Restates | I Explanation | E Question | I Question |
|---|---|---|---|---|
| Event answers | 0 | 0 | 2 | 4 |
| Issue answers | 59 | 12 | 107 | 159 |

| | E CRQ | I CRQ | I Formulation | Continuers | FATs |
|---|---|---|---|---|---|
| Event answers | 0 | 0 | 0 | 0 | 0 |
| Issue answers | 3 | 7 | 24 | 46 | 97 |

| | Responses to Additional Information | | | |
| | I Expansions | I Assertions | Continuers | Questions (I & E) |
|---|---|---|---|---|
| Unsolicited Information | 1 | 0 | 14 | 8 |
| Expansions | 3 | 1 | 107 | 66 |
| Assertions | 4 | 4 | 3 | 11 |
| Continuers | 171 | 11 | 1 | 6 |

*Note.* I = issue relevant; E = event relevant; Elab. = elaborations; CRQ = conditionally relevant question; FATs = freestanding acknowledgment tokens.

elaboration showing that a doctor responded directly to the patient's goal of information seeking. In these data, the more notable responses to embedded questions were direct questions ($n = 2$), continuers ($n = 3$), and solicited answers ($n = 2$). No other function category occurred at least twice. The variability in responses suggests these doctors did not respond uniformly to embedded questions, nor were they particularly responsive to the embedded questions. In only two cases were direct answers given; in other cases, very little information was provided.

Second, in addition to requesting information, information exchange competence also involves identifying how patients and physicians provide information to one another. As noted earlier, patients provided topically relevant answers to doctors' questions (see Table 3, responses to questions). In this sample, patients demonstrate a level of competence in that they provided information to physicians that was on topic. There is a considerable amount of time devoted to patient information giving and the resulting amount of information doctors much processes is vast. Thus, it would seem that after patient answers, doctors have an opportunity to either check their understanding of the solicited information (verifying) or continue on the topic.

In this sample, doctors generally chose to follow up patient issue answers with further questions ($n = 266$, event and issue combined), acknowledge that information with a token ($n = 97$), or verify with restatements and formulations ($n = 83$ combined; see Table 3, responses to answers). What is the better strategy here? Should one verify the information received first and then continue on the topic? Or should one first provide continuers or acknowledgment tokens and then later use formulations for larger chunks of information? These doctors have chosen the latter approach of continuing on the topic and formulating less often. It is unclear if this is the more competent strategy for achieving such goals as understanding information received as well as creating positive relational states.

Relatedly, other ways that physicians and patients attend to unsolicited information provided were examined. Do doctors respond more directly to unsolicited information versus solicited information? In these data, physicians generally did not choose a different strategy for responding to unsolicited information. For instance, after providing unsolicited information, physicians responded with continuers and further questions (see Table 3, responses to additional information). Following patient information with continuers and questions is the same sequence of moves employed when responding to solicited information. There seems no discernable difference in physicians' strategies for responding to patient concerns. Yet, asking issue-relevant questions after unsolicited information seems to be a competent response in that it demonstrates a high level of attention on the physician's part to recognizing new information provided by the other (and potentially useful for diagnosis decisions).

More evidence for the continuer or question response pattern is found in looking at what follows expansions and assertions (other attempts at information giving). Notice in Table 3 that continuers and questions also follow these attempts at information providing. Once the physician gives the continuer prompt, what happens next? Given a continuer, the other participant followed with an expansion 171 times. This pattern suggests more information is provided after a continuer. Based on these data, use of conversational continuers appears to be a moderately competent way of keeping the other person talking on issue relevant topics.

A specific pattern of physician response to patient information seems to emerge from these data. The pattern appears to be information provided → continuer → more information provided. Continuers proved to be a useful information-gathering strategy for physicians (and patients), but with two caveats. First, use of continuers as a single strategy for follow-up on patient concerns seems to be a less competent move—both for meeting physician and patient goals. As the patient keeps talking, prompted by continuers, a physician less skillful at topic control may not be able to direct the interview as effectively. Further, a patient may not provide the most detailed information if he or she thinks the doctor is not really listening. Backchannels such as "uh huh," "yeah," and "go on" provide only a token of feedback.

The second caveat is that consistent use of continuers, and acknowledgment tokens to a lesser degree, could give patients the illusion that their doctors are listening because doctors' prompts to keep talking are continually provided. Ultimately patients will receive little information from the interview, which patients report wanting more of from their physicians (Cegala et al., 1998; Waitzkin, 1985). Therefore, because patients think the doctor is listening to them, postinterview ratings of doctors' relational sensitivity will be higher than information giving. They feel good about the doctor listening to them, but it is not a competent strategy for helping patients meet their informational goals in the end. These findings need further examination in terms of where in the interview continuers are used more effectively. Perhaps one portion of the interview is more appropriate for this strategy than another portion and it may be the case that continuers are not being used as indiscriminately as it appears.

Surprisingly or not, the same pattern emerged regarding patients and their ability to follow up on information provided by physicians. After doctors provided explanations and justifications, patients responded with continuers ($n = 29$) and issue and event questions ($n = 8$), and they chose these moves more than other kinds of direct information verifying moves such as formulations, restatements, and conditionally relevant questions. After those 29 continuers, only 17 elicited further information from physicians. Continuers in this case did provide additional information, but not terribly frequently. A related finding was that patients who used acknowledgment tokens in response to physician information elicited only eight issue explanations from physicians. What seemed to work for patients was to use continuers, and not acknowledgment tokens. Also, these tokens elicited as many event explanations as issue ones suggesting doctors responded on topic and also chose to shift it as well. Although the use of continuers appears to be a competent sequence of talk regarding patients garnering more information and explanations, there was not a high occurrence of this pattern in these data. Other strategies such as patients asking direct questions or using formulations may serve to check understanding and comprehension of information provided, as well as prompt additional feedback and explanations from physicians.

The last criteria of information exchange involves information verifying, and it is clear that both doctors and patients need to be more adept at checking their understanding during the medical interview. Meeting this goal can be identified in moves such as conditionally relevant questions, formulation, restatements, and the like. Doctors report patients are not very good at this task (Cegala et al., 1998) and not surprisingly patients made few attempts to check their understanding. On the other hand, physicians were noted as using proportionally more information-verifying strategies specifically after solicited information from patients. For instance, given an answer to a question (see Table 3, responses to questions), doctors overwhelmingly chose to respond with a freestanding acknowledgment token (97 times), restatements (59 times), continuer (46 times), and finally with formulations (24 times). For competence in checking understanding of information provided, however, it seems that a freestanding acknowledgment token may not be the most competent choice for checking understanding, but it may invite more talk. Future research should give attention to how both doctors and patients verify or check their understanding of information in the medical interview.

Last, although the doctors in this sample used slightly more socioemotional statements than in previous data (Gillotti et al., in press), there are still relatively few relationship-building utterances in these interactions. As others have noted (Cegala, 1997; Roter, 1989) this is an important, yet complex dimension of doctor–patient interactions. McNeilis (1995) found that doctor and patient dyads categorized as more competent on information exchange were the same dyads who demonstrated considerable attention to relational qualities of the interaction, including topic alignment, positivity to one another, humor, and doctors reinforcing their patients. Frequencies of such statements in these data were so low that sequential analysis proved negligible. However, given the importance of this dimension, future research efforts need to examine how both relational and information exchange utterances function interdependently.

## CONCLUSIONS

In this article, I have provided a brief explanation and application of the CACS. The promise of the CACS is its ability to provide assessments of linguistic communication competence at the dyadic level. On the basis of the results of the coding system applied to these data, some conclusions about communication competence in the medical consultation are made here.

### Competence Assessments

Results of this coding scheme provide some insights into health communication processes between physicians and patients regarding their use of specific linguistic strategies for accomplishing various goals. In particular, the use of continuers and other similar strategies by physicians (and patients) were observed as a recurring pattern within information exchange portions of the consultation. This pattern involved responses to information provided and appeared as a sequence of information provided, a continuer, followed by more information provided. Continuers proved to be a useful information-gathering strategy for physicians and patients, but as discussed earlier, it is not a competent pattern in and of itself. Further, it is speculated that this pattern explains findings of patients' concurrent ratings of doctors' competence. Specifically, patient ratings of physician competence would be higher on relational competence but lower on information provision competence. This finding provides further understanding of how and why patients and physicians make certain judgments about communication within the medical consultation. This coding system appears to tap into content, how it is communicated, and how specific sequences of talk lead to more or less competent interactions and judgments of them. Continued work in this area should prove valuable to researchers seeking to relate communication behaviors and other outcomes.

The importance of the finding that continuers and acknowledgment tokens were pervasive in the medical consultation is that doctors and patients are using them somewhat indiscriminately as a dyad. This may provide evidence for identification of more or less competent verbal strategies in this context. In other words, further research could identify those patients and doctors who do not use them indiscriminately and how that pattern relates to ratings of competence. Additionally, these findings are important because both doctor and patient participants were observed using this strategy. Perhaps their perceptions about the effectiveness of certain linguistic strategies for managing the conversation are relatively the same. I note other related conclusions next.

Doctors and patients are still competent at their respective traditional roles. Doctors gather information primarily through direct questions and patients respond with issue relevant solicited information. Another strategy physicians used to control the direction of the interview was observed in topic changes and event shifts. These alignment moves, along with continuers, were used primarily by physicians for meeting their information goals. Interactively, however, they are not as competent at assisting one another in meeting each other's goals. For instance, patients desire more information, and yet doctors in this sample did not respond uniformly with additional information.

Such observations are related to the pattern of continuer or token use in physician follow-up to patient-initiated topics. The use of the continuer sequence was identified as occurring within sections of the consultation when patients provided solicited information and unsolicited information. This sequence leads to patients providing more information, but not for doctors providing additional information or verbally processing information. Additionally, some evidence did emerge that when patients requested additional information (through questions) doctors did not uniformly provide solicited information in return. Further, patients were not as different as their physician counterparts in responding to information provided. They too used continuers, questions, and tokens in response to information provided. Both doctor and patient participants need to be educated in how to competently follow-up when information is provided, through the use of more open-ended questions, elaborations, explanations, and information verifying utterances.

I note two specific conclusions from the application of the CACS to these data. One, doctors and patients used continuers and tokens rather indiscriminately. This does promote further talk (information shared) but they are used more frequently than follow-up questions, formulations, and restatements. So, although information is shared, it's not being processed communicatively. Two, patients think doctors may be listening to them and thus rate them as relationally competent, but in the long run, patients' information needs are not being met (and they don't respond competently themselves). What appears to be occurring is that informational needs are kept fairly separate from relational concerns. That is, doctors and patients pursue those two goals separately in their talk (Roter, 1989).

These results provide some interesting insights into the interactional dynamics of doctor–patient communication during the medical consultation. In particular, it reveals more or less competent communication strategies for meeting information and relational goals. The results give added insight into doctor–patient communication in general but have specific implications for communication skills training. Using this coding scheme, along with competence scales and thought or feeling protocols can help researchers tap more directly into complex communicative processes in the medical consultation. Also just as important, these methods must be grounded in a conceptual framework (Thompson, 1998) to provide more reliable and valid evidence of the importance of interpersonal communicative processes in this context.

## REFERENCES

Bakeman, R., & Quera, V. (1995). *Analyzing interaction: Sequential analysis with SDIS and GSEQ.* New York: Cambridge University Press.

Cegala, D. J. (1997). A study of doctors' and patients' patterns of information exchange and relational communication during a primary care consultation: Implications for communication skills training. *Journal of Health Communication, 2,* 169–194.

Cegala, D. J., Coleman, M. T., & Turner, J. W. (1998). The development and partial assessment of the medical communication competence scale. *Health Communication, 10,* 261–288.

Cegala, D. J., McGee, D. S., & McNeilis, K. S. (1996). Components of patients' and doctors' perceptions of communication competence during a primary care medical interview. *Health Communication, 8,* 1–28.

Cegala, D. J., McNeilis, K. S., McGee, D. S., & Jonas, P. (1995). A study of doctors' and patients' perceptions of information processing and communication competence during the medical interview. *Health Communication, 7,* 179–203.

Cegala, D. J., & Waldron, V. R. (1992). A study of the relationship between communicative performance and conversation participants' thoughts. *Communication Studies, 43,* 105–123.

Gillotti, C., Thompson, T. L., & McNeilis, K. (in press). Communicative competence in the delivery of bad news. *Social Science & Medicine.*

Holsti, O. R. (1969). *Content analysis for the social sciences and humanities.* Reading, MA: Addison-Wesley.

McNeilis, K. S. (1995). *A preliminary investigation of a coding scheme to assess communication competence in the primary care medical interview.* Unpublished doctoral dissertation, Ohio State University, Columbus.

McNeilis, K. S., & Cegala, D. S. (1997, May). *The communication coordination coding scheme.* Paper presented to the Health Communication Division at the Annual International Communication Association Conference, Montreal, Canada.

Roter, D. L. (1989). Which facets of communication have strong effects on outcomes—A meta analysis. In R. Stewart & D. Roter (Eds.), *Communicating with medical patients* (pp. 183–196). Newbury Park, CA: Sage.

Thompson, T. L. (1998). Patient/health professional communication. In L. Jackson & B. K. Duffy (Eds.), *Health communication research: A guide to developments and directions* (pp. 37–56). Westport, CT: Greenwood.

Tracy, K. (1982). On getting the point: Distinguishing "issue" from "events," as aspect of conversational coherence. In M. Burgoon (Ed.), *Communication Yearbook 5* (pp. 278–301). New Brunswick, NJ: Transaction Books.

Waitzkin, H. (1985). Information giving in medical care. *Journal of Health and Social Behavior, 26,* 81–101.

Wiemann, J. M. (1977). A model of communicative competence. *Human Communication Research, 3,* 195–213.

# Patient-Centered Communication Scoring Method Report on Nine Coded Interviews

Leslie Meredith, Moira Stewart, and Judith Belle Brown

*Centre for Studies in Family Medicine*
*The University of Western Ontario*

Based on the patient-centered clinical method (Brown, Weston, & Stewart, 1989; Levenstein, McCracken, McWhinney, Stewart, & Brown, 1986; Stewart, 1995; Weston, Brown, & Stewart, 1989), a method of scoring patient–doctor encounters that were either audiotaped or videotaped was developed. This scoring procedure has several advantages over the commonly used methods (Bales, 1950; Kaplan, Greenfield, & Ware, 1989; Roter, 1977; Roter, Cole, Kern, Barker, & Grayson, 1990; Stewart, 1984): (a) It does not require that the taped interview between the patient and the doctor be transcribed; and (b) it is theory based, that is, it was developed specifically to assess the behaviors of patients and doctors ascribed by the patient-centered clinical method (Stewart, 1995).

The scoring procedure was described fully in a working paper titled "Assessing Communication Between Patients and Doctors: A Manual for Scoring Patient-Centered Communication" (Brown, Stewart, & Tessier, 1995). Interrater reliability of an earlier version of the scoring was established among three raters at $r$ = .687, .835, and .803 (Brown, Stewart, McCracken, McWhinney, & Levenstein, 1986). A more recent study (Stewart et al., 2000), using the current version, established an interrater reliability of .83 and an intrarater reliability of .73. The validity of the scoring procedure was established by a high correlation (.85) with global scores of experienced communication researchers (Stewart et al., 2000).

The measure allows scores to range theoretically from 0 (*not at all patient-centered*) to 100 (*very patient-centered*) communication and includes three main

Requests for reprints should be sent to Moira Stewart, Centre for Studies in Family Medicine, 245–100 Collip Circle, The University of Western Ontario, Research Park, London, Ontario, Canada N6G 4X8. E-mail: moira@julian.uwo.ca

components. The first component, exploring both the disease and illness experience, involves physicians' understanding two conceptualizations of ill health that need to be explored with patients—disease and illness. The second component, understanding the whole person, involves physicians exploring the context of a patient's life setting (e.g., family, work, social supports) and stage of personal development (e.g., life cycle). The third component of the model deals with finding common ground. An effective management plan requires that physicians and patients reach a mutual understanding and mutual agreement in three key areas: the nature of the problems and priorities, the goals of treatment and management, and the roles of the doctor and patient.

## RESULTS OF THE NINE CODED INTERVIEWS

The mean scores of the nine interviews are as follows: exploring both the patient's disease and illness experience, $M = 56.2$, $SD = 21.0$ (Figure 1); integrated understanding of the whole person, $M = 77.8$, $SD = 31.3$ (Figure 2); finding common ground in (a) doctor expressions, $M = 79.9$, $SD = 25.1$ (Figure 3), and in (b) the interaction, $M = 74.1$, $SD = 21.3$ (Figure 4); and the total patient-centered score, $M = 72.3$, $SD = 13.9$ (Figure 5).

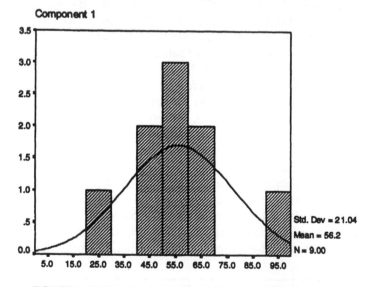

FIGURE 1    Exploring both the patient's disease and illness experience.

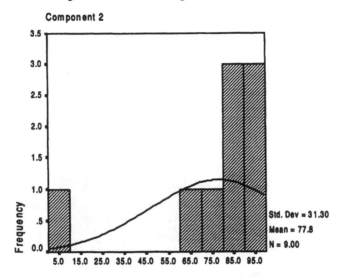

FIGURE 2    Integrated understanding of the whole person.

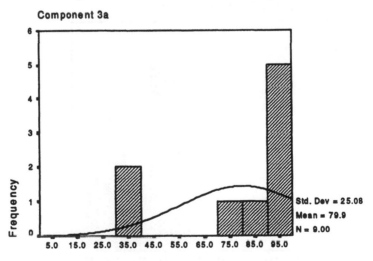

FIGURE 3    Finding common ground in doctor expressions.

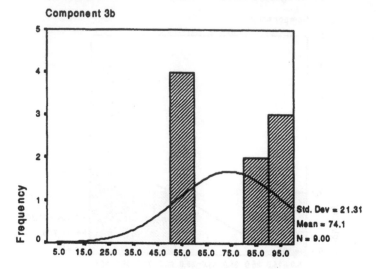

FIGURE 4    Finding common ground in the interaction.

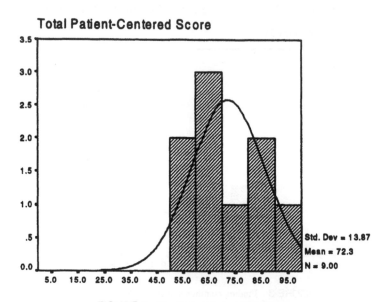

FIGURE 5    The total patient-centered score.

## RESULTS COMPARED TO OTHER STUDIES

The comparison of the results of the nine patient–physician encounters to results of a study of 39 family physicians and 315 patients (Stewart et al., 2000) is shown in Table 1. The 39 family physicians were a random sample of London, Ontario, Canada community-based practitioners with a sample of approximately eight of their patients who visited for a defined list of symptoms. The study's goal was to assess patient-centeredness in relation to patient health outcomes as well as medical care utilization.

Table 1 shows that the distribution for exploring the patient's disease and illness experience (Component 1) was very similar for both this sample and the London, Ontario sample. However, integrated understanding of the whole person (Component 2) was much higher in our sample with a smaller standard deviation. Similarly, finding common ground—doctor expressions and the interaction (Components 3a and 3b)—had a much higher average but their standard deviations were similar.

### Reasons for This Difference in Scores

In this sample, the nine interviews were all with residents. The preceptor entered the room at the end of the interview for each patient, which may have inflated the ratings for both aspects of finding common ground as the two doctors discussed the problem and goals for treatment and management. If the resident had missed or not fully explained the problem(s) and treatment plan, the preceptor often reminded the resident or spoke directly to the patient, resulting in high scores.

TABLE 1
Mean Scores for Each Component of the Patient-Centered Clinical Method

| Components | Current Results[a] | | Patient-Centered Study Results[b] | |
|---|---|---|---|---|
| | M | SD | M | SD |
| 1. Exploring the patient's disease and illness experience | 56.2 | 21.0 | 50.9 | 19.0 |
| 2. Integrated understanding of the whole person | 77.8 | 31.3 | 39.7 | 42.8 |
| 3. Finding common ground | | | | |
| 3a. Doctor expressions | 79.9 | 25.1 | 45.5 | 24.6 |
| 3b. The interaction | 74.1 | 21.3 | 67.1 | 21.3 |
| Total patient-centered score | 72.3 | 13.9 | 50.7 | 17.9 |

[a]$n = 9$. [b]$n = 315$.

Similarly, understanding the whole person may have been artificially inflated. The resident usually completed a checklist of questions designed for new patients that included an exploration of marital status and living arrangements. Due to the nature of the patient-centered scoring method, the resident was awarded a "preliminary exploration" just for inquiring about marital status and, if the doctor pursued the topic by asking one more related question, they received a "further exploration" or, in other words, full marks for this area. Again, due to the nature of the method, if only one topic is explored, and it is explored fully, the entire component will receive full marks. The overall score is calculated by averaging the scores over all components; consequently if scores from one component are inflated, the final patient-centered score will be higher as well.

To conclude, this method of scoring may not be as effective for interviews in which a second physician (in this case a preceptor) is part of the patient encounter due to an artificial inflation of the finding common ground component. Also, those (Stewart et al., 2000) who designed the measure may need to reexamine the scoring of understanding the whole person (Component 2). Completing a checklist that includes some "whole person" questions, is not necessarily congruent with a patient-centered approach.


## RESULTS OF INDIVIDUAL INTERVIEWS

The nine residents can be loosely grouped by low, average, and high scores.

### Exploring the Patient's Disease and Illness Experience (Component 1)

This component has six categorizations: symptoms, prompts, ideas, expectations, feelings, and impact on function. If the physician does not address a patient's statement, a score of 0 is received. If the statement is preliminarily explored with no cutoff, score = 2; if further explored with no cutoff, score = 3. If explored (either preliminary or further) then cut off, score = 1. The score for each category is obtained by averaging the statement scores. The final score is an average of the category scores (see Table 2).

Doctors 3, 7, and 8 received low scores (range = 25–41) for different reasons. Doctors 3 and 8 did not address many of the categories and therefore received a low score. Doctor 7, on the other hand, had discussions in many of the categories but did not explore three (prompts, ideas, impact on function) very completely. Two patient prompts, one idea and the patient's statement about impact on function, were ignored (0 score). This led to a low overall score. The three doctors (1, 9, and 10) who received average scores (range = 53–54) had much the same pattern. Although these doctors on average discussed more of the categories, the explora-

TABLE 2
Score and Number of Statements for Each Interview Categorized by Low, Average, and High Scores

| Doctor No. | Component 1[a] | Component Subscores | | | | | |
|---|---|---|---|---|---|---|---|
| | | Symptom | Prompts | Feeling | Ideas | Function | Expects |
| Low | | | | | | | |
| 3 | 25.0 | 3.0 (3) | — | — | — | — | — |
| 8 | 41.7 | 3.0 (4) | — | — | — | 2.0 (1) | — |
| 7 | 42.8 | 2.7 (7) | 1.0 (3) | — | 1.0 (2) | 0.0 (1) | 3.0 (1) |
| Average | | | | | | | |
| 1 | 54.7 | 2.8 (6) | — | 1.5 (2) | 1.9 (4) | — | 2.0 (1) |
| 9 | 53.7 | 2.67 (3) | 2.0 (1) | — | — | 2.0 (1) | 3.0 (1) |
| 10 | 53.3 | 3.0 (5) | — | — | — | 3.0 (1) | 2.0 (1) |
| High | | | | | | | |
| 2 | 100.0 | 3.0 (5) | — | 3.0 (1) | 3.0 (1) | 3.0 (1) | 3.0 (1) |
| 6 | 65.3 | 3.0 (3) | 1.75 (2) | 2.0 (1) | 0.0 (1) | 3.0 (1) | 2.0 (1) |
| 11 | 68.9 | 2.33 (3) | — | 2.0 (3) | 3.0 (1) | 1.0 (1) | 2.0 (2) |

Note.   The number of statements are in parentheses.
[a]Component 1 = exploring the patient's disease and illness experience.

tion was not complete. For Doctor 1, of the four ideas brought forth by the patient, one was ignored (score of 0) and two received only a preliminary exploration (score of 1), which reduced the score. Doctor 9 explored fewer symptoms, fully exploring two but only preliminarily exploring one. Two other categories only received preliminary exploration. Although Doctor 10 had discussions in fewer categories, he or she fully explored all symptoms and expectations. These two scenarios lead to the average overall score.

The range for the high-score participants (Doctors 2, 6, and 11) is quite wide (65–100). Doctor 2 did an excellent job—having full explorations of five of six categories. As a result, the patient had no need to prompt the physician. Due to the scoring system in which, if patients do not initiate a prompt, the doctor is not penalized, this leads to a perfect score. The interview with Doctors 6 and 11 covered most categories of the scoring system for Component 1. The scores were higher than average but lower than Doctor 2 due to the lack of full explorations in many areas and exploration of expectations was cut off.

## Integrated Understanding of the Whole Person (Component 2)

For this component, the scoring is similar to Component 1. The final score is an average of the statement scores (see Table 3).

TABLE 3
Score and Number of Statements for Each Interview
Categorized by Low, Average, and High Scores

| Doctor No. | Component 2[a] Score | No. of Statements |
|---|---|---|
| Low | | |
| 1 | 66.7 | 3 |
| 11 | 0 | 0 |
| Average | | |
| 2 | 83.3 | 4 |
| 3 | 77.8 | 3 |
| 7 | 83.3 | 2 |
| 9 | 88.9 | 3 |
| High | | |
| 6 | 100.0 | 1 |
| 8 | 100.0 | 3 |
| 10 | 100.0 | 3 |

[a]Component 2 = understanding the whole person.

Only two doctors received scores that could be considered low based on the overall average. Doctor 1 provided only a preliminary exploration (i.e., asked where the patient worked then dropped the subject) of topics related to the patient's personal life. Doctor 11 did not broach any personal subjects during the encounter; it was totally biomedical in nature, thus a score of 0. Each of the average scoring doctors (2, 3, 7, and 9) explored some aspect of the patients' personal life. The reduction in score comes from preliminary exploration of a few statements but, in general, the topics were well covered.

Doctor 6 received a high score by fully exploring one aspect of the patient's personal life. This is a potential problem with the scoring system. For example, Doctor 2, although he or she received an average score, actually fully explored two personal issues yet received a lower score than Doctor 6. This was due to the two other statements being only preliminarily explored. Because the component score is based on the average of scores for each statement, the lower scores reduce the average. Doctors 8 and 10 fully explored all three of the personal issues discussed.

## Finding Common Ground: Doctor Expressions (Component 3a)

For this component, there are two categories: problem definition and goals for treatment and management. Each heading includes two criteria for scoring (yes or no): Was the problem or goal clearly expressed, and did the doctor provide an opportunity to ask questions. One point is awarded for each *yes*. A score of 2 represents full marks for each of the categories (see Table 4).

The low-score participants for this component fell well below the average. Both Doctor 7 and 9 received a low score on this section because they did not define the patient's problem. This is normally done near the end of the interview (e.g., "I think you have a severe muscle pull ...") and is usually followed by the goals for treatment or management plan. In this case, goals for treatment or management were discussed without a clear statement of the problem. This is an important part of the medical encounter as it ensures that the patient understands the exact nature of the health issue. It may be that these doctors assumed the problem was clear, but, without an explicit statement, the patient does not have the opportunity to ask questions about the doctor's diagnosis.

Because the average was very high for this component, the average score participants actually obtained was very good. Doctors 1 and 11 reduced their score by not providing the patient with the opportunity to ask questions for at least one of the goals for treatment or management. Doctor 10 lowered his or her score by not providing the opportunity to ask questions regarding the definition of the problem.

The high-score participants were all above 95 (out of a possible 100). Each of the high-scoring doctors discussed many goals for treatment or management (5–6) with their patients. It is in this section that three of the four doctors reduced their score minimally. Two did not provide opportunity to ask questions on one of the goals and one did not clearly express one of the goals.

TABLE 4
Score and Number of Statements for Each Interview Categorized by Low, Average, and High Scores

| Doctor No. | Problem Definition | Goals for Treatment/ Management | Finding Common Ground Doctor Expressions |
|---|---|---|---|
| Low | | | |
| 7 | 0 (0) | 1.5  (2) | 37.5 |
| 9 | 0 (0) | 1.5  (4) | 37.5 |
| Average | | | |
| 1 | 2 (1) | 1.56 (9) | 89.0 |
| 10 | 1 (1) | 2.0  (4) | 75.0 |
| 11 | 2 (1) | 1.75 (4) | 93.8 |
| High | | | |
| 2 | 2 (1) | 1.83 (6) | 95.8 |
| 3 | 2 (1) | 1.83 (6) | 95.8 |
| 6 | 2 (1) | 1.8  (5) | 95.8 |
| 8 | 2 (2) | 2.0  (5) | 100.0 |

*Note.*    The number of statements are in parentheses.

## Finding Common Ground: The Interaction (Component 3b)

For this component, there are two main categories: problem definition and goals for treatment or management, and a third category, responded to disagreement with flexibility, which is scored only if a disagreement occurs. Each category includes two criteria for scoring (*yes* or *no*): mutual discussion and clarification of agreement. A score of 2 represents full marks for each category (see Table 5).

Four of the 9 participants did not score well on this component. Doctor 1 received a lower score by partially discussing both the problem definition and goals for treatment or management. The other low-scoring doctors did a good job on the goals for treatment or management but did not define the problem at all. Therefore, Doctors 7 and 9 received a 0 score. On the other hand, although Doctor 10 had defined the problem under doctor expressions, he or she did not allow for a mutual discussion or clarification of agreement on the defined problem. This is central to the patient and physician finding common ground and, if not done, can lead to problems of nonadherence to treatment.

The average scores were actually very good scores overall. Doctors 2 and 11 did not mutually discuss or obtain clarification of agreement for one of the statements discussed although all others were done well. Doctor 8 did not obtain clarification of agreement for one of the health problems discussed. If a patient does not explicitly have the opportunity to agree or disagree with a diagnosis, there is a greater likelihood of lack of adherence to treatment. In the patient encounter with Doctor 8, a disagreement occurred over one of the suggested treat-

TABLE 5
Score and Number of Statements for Each Interview Categorized by Low, Average, and High Scores

| Doctor No. | Problem Definition | Goals for Treatment/ Management | Responded to Disagreement With Flexibility[a] | Finding Common Ground Interaction |
|---|---|---|---|---|
| Low |
| 1 | 1.0 (1) | 1.33 (9) | — | 58.3 |
| 7 | 0 (0) | 2.0  (2) | — | 50.0 |
| 9 | 0 (0) | 2.0  (4) | — | 50.0 |
| 10 | 0 (1) | 2.0  (4) | — | 50.0 |
| Average |
| 2 | 2.0 (1) | 1.5  (6) | — | 87.5 |
| 8 | 1.5 (2) | 2.0  (5) | 2 (1) | 91.7 |
| 11 | 2.0 (1) | 1.5  (4) | — | 87.5 |
| High |
| 3 | 2.0 (1) | 1.83 (6) | 2 (1) | 97.2 |
| 6 | 2.0 (1) | 1.8  (5) | — | 95.0 |

*Note.*  The number of statements are in parentheses.
[a]Only scored in the event that a disagreement arose.

TABLE 6
Score for Each Interview Categorized by Low, Average, and High Scores

| Doctor No. | Patient Centered | Understanding the Disease and Illness Experience | Understanding the Whole Person | Finding Common Ground | |
|---|---|---|---|---|---|
| | | | | Doctor Expressions | The Interaction |
| Low | | | | | |
| 7 | 53.4 | 42.8 (L) | 83.3 (A) | 37.5 (L) | 50.0 (L) |
| 9 | 57.5 | 53.7 (A) | 88.9 (A) | 37.5 (L) | 50.0 (L) |
| 11 | 62.6 | 68.9 (H) | 0 (L) | 93.8 (A) | 87.5(A) |
| Average | | | | | |
| 1 | 67.2 | 54.7 (A) | 66.7 (L) | 89.0 (A) | 58.3 (L) |
| 3 | 74.0 | 25.0 (L) | 77.8 (A) | 95.8 (H) | 97.2 (H) |
| 10 | 69.6 | 53.3 (A) | 100.0 (H) | 75.0 (A) | 50.0 (L) |
| High | | | | | |
| 2 | 91.7 | 100.0 (H) | 83.3 (A) | 95.8 (H) | 87.5 (A) |
| 6 | 88.8 | 65.3 (H) | 100.0 (H) | 95.0 (H) | 95.0 (H) |
| 8 | 85.9 | 41.7 (L) | 100.0 (H) | 100.0 (H) | 91.7 (A) |

*Note.*  L = low score; A = average score; H = high score.

ments. In this case the physician responded with flexibility to the disagreement by respecting the patient's wishes while explaining the possible consequences, hence the score of 2.

Doctors 3 and 6 did an excellent job on this component. They clearly expressed the problem, provided an opportunity to ask questions, promoted mutual discussion, and obtained agreement on the goals for treatment or management.

## Total Patient-Centered Score

Table 6 shows the total patient scores for each interview. Two of the low-scoring doctors scored poory on the finding common ground section of the patient-centered method. This suggests that the patient and doctor did not come to a mutual understanding of the problems identified during the visit. This lack of common ground could lead to lack of adherence to treatment or medication regimens, or both. It also may inhibit the building of a productive patient–doctor relationship due to the patient not feeling he or she was part of the decision-making process. One doctor did not explore personal issues (understanding the whole person). This component is central to the patient-centered method in that the patient's life context is important to understanding the patient and may impact on treatment decisions. The average-scoring doctors each did well but had particular areas in which they could improve. Full explorations of all topics would have increased their scores and resulted in a more patient-centered interview. The interview by Doctor 2 could be used as an example for doctors who wish to practice patient-centered medicine. The other two high-scoring doctors did very well but could improve their scores on understanding the whole person or understanding the disease and illness experience, or both. These are areas that need to be developed in a truly patient-centered interview.

## SUMMARY AND CONCLUSIONS

In summary, the 9 participants received high patient-centered scores based on this measure of communication that assesses the degree of patient-centeredness during a single encounter with a patient. However, there are limitations as the sample consisted of only nine physicians with a single patient. In addition, the participants were residents and during each encounter the preceptor joined the doctor and patient at the conclusion of the encounter, which, as we previously noted, may have inflated the scores based on this measure. Some limitations of the measure have also been identified. For example, when a physician conducts a checklist of patient's personal demographics (e.g., marital status, employment) these are considered under Component 2, understanding the whole person. Yet, this does not reflect an integrated understanding of the whole person. Clearly, adjustments to this component of the measure are required. A second observation is that the presence of a third person in the encounter alters the scoring procedure. In this case it was the preceptor but the presence of a patient caregiver could similarly alter the scoring process. Finally, this scoring mechanism of averaging the number of symptoms, ideas, and so forth presented by the patient and ultimately explored by the physician requires review.

## REFERENCES

Bales, R. F. (1950). *Interaction process analysis: A method for the study of small groups.* Reading, MA: Addison-Wesley.

Brown, J. B., Stewart, M. A., McCracken, E. C., McWhinney, I. R., & Levenstein, J. H. (1986). The patient-centered clinical method: 2. Definition and application. *Family Practice: An International Journal, 3,* 75–79.

Brown, J. B., Stewart, M., & Tessier, S. (1995). *Assessing communication between patients and doctors: A manual for scoring patient-centered communication* (Working paper series, Paper No. 95–2). London, Canada: University of Western Ontario, Centre for Studies in Family Medicine.

Brown, J. B., Weston, W. W., & Stewart, M. A. (1989). Patient-centered interviewing: Pt. 2. Finding common ground. *Canadian Family Physician, 35,* 153–157.

Kaplan, S. H., Greenfield, S., & Ware, J. E. (1989). Assessing the effects of physician–patient interactions on the outcomes of chronic disease. *Medical Care, 275,* 5110–5127.

Levenstein, J. H., McCracken, E. C., McWhinney, I. R., Stewart, M. A., & Brown, J. B. (1986). The patient-centered clinical method: 1. A model for the doctor–patient interaction in family medicine. *Family Practice: An International Journal, 3,* 24–30.

Roter, D. L. (1977). Patient participation in patient–provider interaction: The effects of patient question-asking on the quality of interaction, satisfaction, and compliance. *Health Education Monographs, 5,* 281–315.

Roter, D. L., Cole, K. A., Kern, D. E., Barker, L. R., & Grayson, M. (1990). An evaluation of residency training in interviewing skills and the psychosocial domain of medical practice. *Journal of General Internal Medicine, 28,* 375–388.

Stewart, M. A. (1984). What is a successful doctor–patient interview? A study of interactions and outcomes. *Social Science & Medicine, 19,* 167–175.

Stewart, M. (1995). Effective physician–patient communication and health outcomes: A review. *Canadian Medical Association Journal, 152,* 1423–1433.

Stewart, M., Brown, J. B., Donner, A., McWhinney, I. R., Oates, J., Weston, W., & Jordan, J. (2000). The impact of patient-centered care on outcomes. *The Journal of Family Practice, 49,* 796–804.

Weston, W. W., Brown, J. B., & Stewart, M. A. (1989). Patient-centered interviewing: Pt. 1. Understanding patients' experiences. *Canadian Family Physician, 35,* 147–151.

# The Relationship Between Residents' and Attending Physicians' Communication During Primary Care Visits: An Illustrative Use of the Roter Interaction Analysis System

Debra L. Roter and Susan Larson

*Department of Health Policy and Management*
*Johns Hopkins School of Public Health*

The medical dialogue is the fundamental instrument by which the doctor–patient relationship is crafted and by which problem solving and decision making regarding medical management and therapeutic goals are accomplished. Derived loosely from social exchange theories related to interpersonal influence, problem solving (Bales, 1950; Emerson, 1976), and reciprocity (Ben-Sira, 1976; Davis, 1969; Gouldner, 1960; Roter & Hall, 1989), the Roter Interaction Analysis System (RIAS; Roter, 1999) provides a tool for viewing the dynamics and consequences of patients' and providers' exchange of resources through the interaction of the medical dialogue. The social exchange orientation is consistent with health education and empowerment perspectives that view the medical encounter as a "meeting between experts" grounded in an egalitarian model of patient–provider partnership that rejects expert-domination and passive-patient roles (Freire, 1983; Roter, 1987, 2000a, 2000b; Roter & Hall, 1991; Tuckett, Boulton, Olson, & Williams, 1985; Wallerstein & Bernstein, 1988).

RIAS categories can be broadly viewed as reflecting socioemotional and task-focused elements of medical exchange. Physicians' *task-focused behaviors* are defined as technically based skills used in problem solving that comprise the base of the expertise for which a physician is consulted (Ben-Sira, 1980; Parsons,

Requests for reprints should be sent to Debra L. Roter, Department of Health Policy and Management, Johns Hopkins School of Public Health, 624 North Broadway, Baltimore, MD 21205. E-mail: droter@jhsph.edu

1951). Task behaviors include such things as the choice of diagnostic tests, as well as the conduct of procedures such as drawing blood, giving injections, and performing a physical exam. The value of these activities, however, is limited without the talk that organizes and informs the history and puts symptoms, treatment, and management in a meaningful context for both patients and physicians.

From a communication perspective, physicians' task behaviors include data gathering and patient education and counseling within both the biomedical and psychosocial domains. The affective dimension of physician behavior includes verbal exchanges with explicit socioemotional content related to the building of social and emotional rapport. Affect may also be conveyed implicitly through tone of voice or through a general impression of positive (friendliness or interest) or negative emotion (anxiety or irritation). Patient behaviors can be seen in a parallel manner with information giving and question asking, both biomedical and psychosocial, in the task domain and social conversation; approvals or disagreements; and statements of concern in the affective domain (Hall, Roter, & Katz, 1987).

Although the underlying theoretical structure was drawn from the work cited previously, face validity of the RIAS's capture of the primary elements of medical exchange is provided by a meta-analysis of communication studies (Hall, Roter, & Katz, 1988; Roter, Hall, & Katz, 1988). The meta-analysis undertook an exhaustive review of published studies in which audio or video of medical communication was analyzed. Over 250 different elements of communication were identified in the 61 studies reviewed. This list was reduced to four primary communication categories (and one category reflecting judgments of technical and interpersonal competence): information giving, question asking, partnership building, and socioemotional behaviors. The RIAS includes these categories in elaborated detail, as well as several other less frequently investigated communication elements, providing confidence that it captures the fundamental elements of medical exchange common to most analytic systems.

The RIAS system has been widely used in studies in the United States and Europe and has been applied to a variety of medical settings and specialties as both a descriptive and evaluative research and teaching tool. It has been used to describe communication in adult and pediatric primary care, emergency medicine; specialty care including obstetrics and gynecology, oncology, surgery, nursing, podiatry, and dentistry, as well as to evaluate medical training and continuing medical education programs, and predict patient and physician outcomes. (See the Appendix bibliography that lists selected RIAS-related studies by outcome or emphasis.)

In the context of our study, RIAS analysis has been applied to 10 audiotapes of medical visits between patients and their medical residents. In 8 of these visits, an attending physician was present and consulted with the resident about the case for varying periods of time. We were intrigued by the variation in the communication profiles of attending physicians in the visits and therefore structured our analysis to explore the relation between residents' and attending physicians' communication during these medical encounters.

The specific objectives of the analysis are threefold: (a) to describe the communication profiles of the primary care residents and their patients using the RIAS, (b) to describe the communication profiles of attending physicians assisting the residents during these visits using the RIAS, and (c) to explore the relation between variation in attending physicians' communication profile and the communication characteristics of the residents and their patients.

## METHOD

A useful framework for organizing and grounding RIAS-coded communication in the clinical encounter is the functional model of medical interviewing (Cohen-Cole, 1991; Lazare, Putnam, & Lipkin, 1995) as displayed in Table 1. Task behaviors fall within two of the medical interview functions: *gathering data* to understand the patient's problems and *educating and counseling* patients about their illness and motivating patients to adhere to treatment. Affective behaviors generally reflect the third medical interview function of *building a relationship* through the development of rapport and responsiveness to the patient's emotions. A fourth function of the visit can be added: *activating and partnership building,* to enhance patients' capacity to engage in an effective partnership with their physician. Although not explicitly defined by the authors of the functional model, the use of verbal strategies to help patients integrate, synthesize, and translate between the biomedical and psychosocial paradigms of the therapeutic dialogue deserves special note. The activating function facilitates the expression of patients' expectations, preferences, and perspectives so that they may more meaningfully participate in treatment and management decision making (Roter, 2000b).

The RIAS is applied to the smallest unit of expression or statement to which a meaningful code can be assigned, generally a complete thought, expressed by each speaker throughout the medical dialogue. These units are assigned to mutually exclusive and exhaustive categories that reflect the content and form of the medical dialogue. Form distinguishes statements that are primarily informative (information giving), persuasive (counseling), interrogative (closed- and open-ended questions), affective (social, positive, negative, and emotional), and process oriented (participatory facilitators, orientations, and transitions). In addition to form, content areas are specified for exchanges about medical condition and history, therapeutic regimen, lifestyle behaviors, and psychosocial topics relating to social relations and feelings and emotions.

In addition to the verbal categories of exchange, coders rate each speaker on a 6-point scale reflecting a range of affective dimensions including anger, anxiety, dominance, interest, and friendliness. These ratings have been found to reflect

TABLE 1
Categories of the Roter Interaction Analysis System (Roter, 1999)

| Functional Grouping | Communication Behavior | Examples |
|---|---|---|
| Patient education and counseling | Biomedical information-giving (medical condition, therapeutic regimen) | The medication may make you drowsy. You need it for 10 days. |
| | Psychosocial information-giving (lifestyle, self-care information) | The community center is good for company and you can get meals there. |
| | Biomedical counseling (persuasive statements regarding medical management and therapeutic regimen) | Its important to take those pills everyday, I don't want you to miss any. Watch that foot for infection, be sure to keep it clean and you won't have a problem. |
| | Psychosocial counseling (persuasive statements regarding lifestyle changes and social psychological issues) | Getting exercise is a good idea, especially now. The most important thing you can do is just quit—just do it! It's important to get out and do something with someone every day. |
| Data gathering | Open-ended questions: medical (medical condition, therapeutic regimen) | What can you tell me about the pain? How are the meds working? |
| | Open-ended questions: psychosocial (lifestyle, social psychological) | What are you doing to keep yourself healthy? What's happening with your father? |
| | Closed-ended questions: medical (medical condition, therapeutic regimen) | Does it hurt now? Are you taking your meds? |
| | Closed-ended questions: psychosocial (lifestyle, social psychological) | Are you still smoking? Is your wife back? |
| Building a relationship | Social talk (nonmedical chitchat) | How about them Os last night? |
| | Positive talk (agreements, jokes, approvals, laughter) | You look fantastic, you are doing great. |
| | Negative talk (disagreements, criticisms) | I think you are wrong, you weren't being careful. No, I do want that. |
| | Emotional talk (concerns, reassurance, empathy, partnership) | I'm worried about that. I'm sure it will get better. We'll get through this. |
| Activating and partnering | Participatory facilitators (asking for patient opinion, asking for understanding, paraphrases, back channels) | What do you think it is? Do you follow me? I heard you say you didn't like that. Let me make sure I've got it right. … Uh-huh, right, go on, hmm. |
| | Procedural talk (orientations, transitions) | I'll first look at your rash and then take your blood pressure. I'll be back in a minute. Well, OK. Now … |

voice tone channels that are largely independent of literal verbal content (Hall, Roter, & Rand, 1981).

The system is flexible and responsive to study context by adding or elaborating tailored categories. Coders may also mark the phases of the visit so that the opening, history segment, physical exam, counseling and discussion segment, and closing are specified and communication falling within these parts of the visit can be analyzed and summarized separately (e.g., Roter, Lipkin, & Korsgaard, 1991). Depending on the question of interest, coders may be asked to make a variety of qualitative notations, selected verbatim transcription, or rating of skill use or targeted behaviors, for later analysis or reporting (e.g., Crain et al., 1999).

Because the unit of analysis is the smallest unit of expression or statement to which a meaningful code can be assigned, and these are mutually exclusive and exhaustive, the RIAS codes can be considered building blocks or basic communication elements that can be used individually or combined to summarize the dialogue in a variety of ways. Table 1 displays the individual categories and examples of some of the larger variable composites derived from them. For instance, within the data-gathering function, open- and closed-ended questions across content areas are specified allowing for analysis of individual question-asking variables as well as a variety of permutations, including all medical questions or psychosocial questions (open and closed), all open- or closed-ended questions (biomedical and psychosocial), a ratio of open to closed questions (over biomedical, psychosocial, or all topics), or a ratio of biomedical to psychosocial questions (over closed-ended or open-ended questions). Similar groupings can be derived from information giving and counseling categories. Other variable combinations representing composites of partnership building, emotional talk, and positive talk are also displayed in Table 1.

In addition to variable combinations, other calculations can be made, including total amount of talk (by participant), ratios of provider to patient talk as an indication of verbal dominance, and proportion of biomedical to psychosocial talk as a reflection of topic focus. Patient-centeredness scores can be computed by calculating a ratio of patient versus physician communication control—the sum of physician information giving (including both biomedical and psychosocial) and patient psychosocial information giving and question asking divided by the sum of physician question asking and patient biomedical information giving. This is similar to the approach taken in several of our own studies (Roter et al., 1997; Wissow et al., 1998) and by other investigators (Ford, Fallowfield, & Lewis, 1996; Greenfield, Kaplan, & Ware, 1985; Mead & Bower, 2000).

The RIAS code definitions are straightforward, intuitive, and easily learned. Training is accomplished over a 3-day period with acceptable levels of reliability and speed generally achieved with several weeks of practice. Experienced RIAS coders average 50% over real time for an uncomplicated coding task; a 30-min visit can be expected to be coded in less than 45 min. Coders apply the RIAS directly to audiotapes without transcription, using direct-entry software that can be applied to digitized audio or video files or used with analogue audiotape or video-tape recordings. When additional coding tasks are added, for instance noting the presence of targeted skills, adding selected verbatim excerpts of dialogue or word use, or marking the dialogue of additional participants, coding time may be longer.

The RIAS demonstrates good reliability; Pearson correlation coefficients average well over .85 for high-frequency categories and above .70 for categories with less than one occurrence per encounter. Effective reliabilities for grouped variables are well over .90.

## RESULTS

The average length of visit is 32 min; ranging widely from 19 to 54 min. Attendings participated in eight of these visits, but for relatively short time periods. On average, attendings were verbally active for 4.6 min, but this input varied from 1.6 min to slightly over 8 min. The number of statements made by the residents averaged 375 with a wide range (166–706), reflecting the variation already noted in the length of visit. Attending physicians contributed an average of 41 statements (range = 5–104). Patients were less verbally active than residents, averaging 285 statements (range = 176–511). The relative contribution of each speaker to the medical dialogue can be represented by a simple ratio of speaker to speaker talk. The ratio of resident to patient talk averages 1.3:1 (with a range from less than 1:1 to almost 2:1). These ratios can be viewed as a gross indicator of verbal dominance.

In a similar vein, a ratio of resident to attending talk can be calculated. As expected, residents are the dominant speaker with an average ratio of 17:1 relative to the attending physicians' contribution to the dialogue. Most interesting in this light are three visits in which the ratio was quite small (between 2:1 and 5:1) reflecting a relatively high contribution by the attending. The relation between the total length of visit and amount of attending time in the room was not significant (Pearson $r =$ .29, $p < .5$); indeed, the visit in which the attending spent the longest period of time with his or her resident (8 min) was 30.5 min, very close to the sample mean, whereas the shortest period of attending time (1.6 min) was associated with a slightly higher than mean length of visit (36.4 min).

Although the length of visit and amount of talk are correlated, they are not entirely redundant measures. In this sample, for instance, the total length of visit (in seconds) is highly correlated with both physician and patient talk (Pearson $r$ = .90 and .80, $p < .005$, respectively). Indeed, the frequency of patient and physician talk is highly correlated (Pearson $r = .81$, $p < .005$). The correlation between length of time the attending is present and total amount of attending talk is slightly weaker than for the primary speakers, although still significant (Pearson $r = .70$, $p < .05$).

## Resident and Attending Profile of Interaction

Table 2 displays the profile of communication for both residents and attendings across the four functions of the visit, as described earlier. The visit emphasis is clearly biomedical as evidenced by the distribution across content areas in the two most prominent exchange categories, education and counseling and data gathering. Patient education and counseling accounts for 20% of resident talk; 19% of this is devoted to biomedical topics. Half of this discussion is devoted specifically to information giving about the therapeutic regimen, and the rest is about equally divided between information about the patient's medical condition and persuasive counseling regarding medical and treatment issues. Lifestyle and psychosocial topic discussion and counseling accounts for less than 2% of residents' talk.

Data gathering is the single largest category used by residents and accounts for almost one fourth of all resident talk. The table shows that about 80% of these questions are closed-ended and 80% are about biomedical topics. It is notable that although physicians appear reticent about giving information or counseling in the lifestyle or psychosocial realm, they are somewhat less so in making inquiries into these topics. Lifestyle and psychosocial questions account for 20% of all data gathering attempts.

Positive responses to patient statements are frequent and comprise 20% of resident talk. These are mostly agreements indicating acceptance of patient statements, but also include laughter and jokes, and statements of approval. Consistent with the biomedical focus of the visits, only 5% of resident talk is explicitly related to patient emotions. Within this domain, the most frequent element of talk is reassurance, followed by concern statements.

Activating and partnering comprises 16% of resident talk, mostly by paraphrase and interpretation and verbal indicators of attention. Finally, related to partnering, residents devote about 14% of talk to providing the patient with orientations and transitions, which are cues to what is expected of them and what will be happening next in the visit.

Differences in the communication profile distributions between residents and attendings are evident in all four of the visit functions—education and counseling, data gathering, rapport building, and providing procedural cues to the patient. Table 2 also shows these distributions. Attending physicians engage in more biomedical education than residents, with most of this devoted to information about the therapeutic regimen. They ask proportionately fewer questions than residents overall, but with more questions devoted to biomedical relative to psychosocial topics. In the rapport-building domain, attendings engage in a substantially higher proportion of social talk than residents, although in raw numbers this may simply reflect an introduction and greeting, and slightly higher percentages of emotional talk. Finally, residents provide substantially more orientations and directions to their patients than do the attending physicians and about the same amount of activating and partnering.

TABLE 2
Communication Categories Used by Residents and Attendings

| Category | Resident Talk | | | Attending Talk | | |
|---|---|---|---|---|---|---|
| | M | Range | % | M | Range | % |
| Education and counseling | | | | | | |
|   Biomedical topics | 70.9 | 28–123 | 18.9 | 12.6 | 0–47 | 30.7 |
|     Medical condition | 18.4 | 2–40 | | 3.3 | 0–9 | |
|     Therapeutic regimen | 38.5 | 5–105 | | 8.4 | 0–37 | |
|     Counseling | 14.0 | 2–33 | | 0.9 | 0–5 | |
|   Psychosocial topics | 5.3 | 0–10 | 1.4 | 0.7 | 0–4 | 1.7 |
|     Lifestyle | 3.0 | 0–9 | | 0.4 | 0–2 | |
|     Psychosocial | 0.2 | 0–1 | | 0.1 | 0–1 | |
|     Counseling | 2.1 | 0–9 | | 0.2 | 0–1 | |
| Data gathering | | | | | | |
|   Biomedical questions | 67.7 | 38–132 | 18.1 | 5.5 | 1–14 | 13.4 |
|     Closed-ended | 53.1 | 30–91 | | 5.3 | 1–13 | |
|     Open questions | 14.6 | 6–42 | | 0.2 | 0–1 | |
|   Psychosocial questions | 17.2 | 4–32 | 4.6 | 1.3 | 0–5 | 3.2 |
|     Closed-ended | 12.4 | 3–26 | | 0.7 | 0–3 | |
|     Open questions | 4.8 | 1–11 | | 0.6 | 0–2 | |
| Building a relationship | | | | | | |
|   Social talk | 0.7 | 0–2 | 0.2 | 1.0 | 0–3 | 2.4 |
|   Positive talk | 77.6 | 18–154 | 20.7 | 8.0 | 0–23 | 19.5 |
|     Agreements | 67.2 | 16–148 | | 6.5 | 0–15 | |
|     Approvals | 3.2 | 0–12 | | 0.4 | 0–1 | |
|     Compliments | 0.4 | 0–3 | | 0.5 | 0–1 | |
|     Laughter/jokes | 6.8 | 1–20 | | 0.6 | 0–4 | |
|   Negative talk | 0 | 0–1 | 0 | | | |
|   Emotional talk | 21.5 | 1–71 | 5.7 | 3.4 | 0–10 | 8.3 |
|     Empathy | 0.6 | 0–2 | | 0.3 | 0–2 | |
|     Concern | 6.2 | 0–27 | | 1.0 | 0–7 | |
|     Reassurance | 13.4 | 0–39 | | 2.0 | 0–8 | |
|     Partnership | 0.3 | 0–2 | | 0 | | |
|     Self-disclosure | 0.3 | 0–1 | | 0 | | |
|     Asking for reassurance | 0.7 | 0–2 | | 0 | | |
| Activating and partnering | | | | | | |
|   Participatory facilitators | 60.0 | 24–175 | 16.0 | 5.2 | 0–16 | 12.7 |
|     Back channels | 17.0 | 2–95 | | 1.2 | 0–5 | |
|     Paraphrase | 31.0 | 13–71 | | 3.0 | 0–9 | |
|     Asks for opinion | 1.0 | 0–3 | | 0.4 | 0–2 | |
|     Asks if understood | 10.0 | 1–51 | | 0.6 | 0–5 | |
|     Asks for reassurance | 1.0 | 0–3 | | 0 | | |
|   Procedural talk | 54.0 | 16–87 | 14.4 | 3.0 | 0–7 | 7.3 |
|     Orientations | 28.0 | 9–46 | | 1.8 | 0–6 | |
|     Transitions | 23.0 | 3–42 | | 1.2 | 0–3 | |
|     Procedural questions and information | 3.0 | 0–22 | | 0 | | |
| Uninterpretable[a] | 12.0 | 0–28 | | 1.0 | 0–5 | |

[a]Not included in percentages.

## Patient Profile of Interaction

Table 3 displays the patient distribution of communication elements in parallel manner to that of residents and attendings. Not surprisingly, we see the predominant biomedical focus of the visit reflected in the patient categories. Fully four times as much patient disclosure is in the biomedical realm than the psychosocial realm (53% vs. 12%). Aside from providing information to the resident, most of what is said by patients is positive, in the sense of acknowledgment and agreement. These comprise over 21% of patient exchanges. As was true in the high proportion of physician agreements with patients, these statements mark acknowledgment of physician comments, rather than true agreement with substantive points. About 6% of patient talk is within the explicitly emotional domain, primarily statements of concern.

TABLE 3
Communication Categories Used by Patients

| Category | M | Range | % |
|---|---|---|---|
| Information-giving | | | |
| Biomedical information | 151.0 | 77–313 | 53.0 |
| Medical condition | 125.0 | 70–299 | |
| Therapeutic regimen | 25.0 | 7–55 | |
| Psychosocial information | 34.0 | 12–78 | 11.9 |
| Lifestyle | 30.0 | 12–78 | |
| Psychosocial | 4.0 | 0–13 | |
| Question asking | | | |
| All questions | 3.3 | 0–11 | 1.2 |
| Biomedical questions | 2.8 | 0–11 | |
| Psychosocial questions | 0.5 | 0–2 | |
| Building a relationship | | | |
| Social talk | 1.0 | 0–5 | 0.4 |
| Positive talk | 60.0 | 37–98 | 21.0 |
| Agreements | 47.0 | 16–148 | |
| Approvals | 1.0 | 0–2 | |
| Compliments | 0.0 | 0–4 | |
| Laughter/jokes | 11.0 | 3–30 | |
| Negative talk | 1.0 | 0–4 | 0.4 |
| Emotional talk | 18.5 | 2–110 | 6.5 |
| Empathy | 0.0 | 0–2 | |
| Concern | 17.0 | 1–102 | |
| Reassurance | 1.0 | 0–5 | |
| Facilitators | 3.0 | 0–6 | 1.1 |
| Procedural talk | 13.0 | 0–39 | 4.6 |
| Uninterpretable | 12.0 | 2–39[a] | |

[a]Not included in percentages.

As is evident in many studies, patients ask few questions; only 1% of their talk falls within this category. Other specific categories of interest include a low frequency of social talk (0.4%) and disagreements (0.4%).

Particular elements of communication are highly reciprocal between patients and physicians. The strongest of these patterns is evident for emotional talk, in which the correlation between patient and resident expression is very high (Pearson $r = .86$, $p < .0001$). Social exchanges are also substantially correlated (Pearson $r = .56$, $p < .09$). Positive talk is primarily acknowledgment of information; this explains the correlation between residents' biomedical information giving and patient positive talk ($.60$, $p < .07$) and patients' biomedical information giving and resident positive talk ($.75$, $p < .01$). There is little relation between patient and residents' positive exchanges ($.01$, $p < .97$).

Patient responses to resident questions is interesting from a reciprocal perspective. Open- and closed-ended biomedical questions elicited significant levels of patients' biomedical disclosure ($.76$, $p < .01$, and $.85$, $p < .002$, respectively); however, open biomedical questions were also significantly correlated with patients' psychosocial disclosure ($.74$, $p < .01$). Psychosocial questions were strongly correlated with patients' psychosocial disclosure, with open questions associated with slightly stronger correlations than closed questions ($.82$, $p < .003$, and $.71$, $p < .02$, respectively). Psychosocial questions, however, were not related to patients' giving of biomedical information to the resident. Residents' use of participatory facilitators was correlated with patient disclosure of both biomedical ($.72$, $p < .01$) and psychosocial information giving ($.67$, $p < .03$) and patient question asking ($.57$, $p < .09$).

In a three-way interaction it is difficult to determine who is the intended target of communication. In this regard the pattern of correlations among communication elements is helpful. Attending physicians' biomedical information giving was related to patients' use of positive talk ($.75$, $p < .03$), indicating that patients perceived the information as directed toward them. Unlike the relation between residents' use of participatory facilitators and patient talk, attendings' facilitators were unrelated to patients' questions or information giving. There was, however, a relation between attendings' use of participatory facilitators and resident talk; the more facilitators attendings used, the less likely residents were to engage in psychosocial exchanges with patients ($-.82$, $p < .001$). This might suggest that the facilitators were primarily targeted toward the residents, rather than the patients.

## Comparison to Communication Patterns of Primary Care Physicians

A useful frame of reference for interpreting the results presented in Tables 2 and 3 is provided by a previous study of primary care visits (Roter et al., 1997). In that study, 127 primary care physicians and 534 of their chronic disease patients were audiotaped to explore the extent to which patterns of communication that relate to ideal relationship types as described in the literature could be identified. Cluster analysis of communication elements revealed five distinct patterns of communication ranging from medically dominated to consumerist in nature. Two medically dominated patterns, each accounting for one third of the visits, warrant special attention within the context of the current analysis.

The first of these was defined as *narrowly biomedical* and was characterized by physician talk that had a high proportion of closed-ended medical questior• (19%), biomedical information giving (27%), and negligible psychosocial exchange (2%). The predominant category of patient talk was biomedical information giving (70%) with little psychosocial disclosure (5%) and few questions. A second, but somewhat *expanded biomedical* pattern of exchange was also identified. The expanded and narrow patterns were similar in high medical questioning (17%) and biomedical information (22%), although the expanded pattern was broader in its inclusion of psychosocial discussion from the doctor (7%). Patient talk was also more evenly spread between biomedical (56%) and psychosocial (16%) topics in the expanded compared with narrow biomedical patterns.

The profile of resident exchanges looks quite a bit like the biomedical expanded pattern, with the resident's psychosocial contribution at about 7% and 12% patient talk coded as psychosocial in nature. Although on average attendings contributed only a small portion of the dialogue, their communication patterns appear more biomedically narrow than that of the residents. The attendings contribution was proportionately more biomedical and less psychosocial in both the patient education and data gathering domains than that of residents. Moreover, the more verbally active the attending was in the visit, the less psychosocial the resident was. The total amount of attending talk was related to psychosocial and emotional elements of the resident's communication style. Regression analysis found that attendings are more verbally active (total of all statements) in visits with residents who engage in less psychosocial talk and less emotional talk with their patients ($R^2$ = .85; standardized $\beta$ = −.95 and −.74, respectively).

## DISCUSSION

The medical visits analyzed for this study were complicated and diverse. The substantive medical problems ranged from management of chronic disease, to multiple injuries, to the first prenatal visit. The variation contributed by patients, medical conditions, residents, and attendings all further complicate the analysis, especially with a sample size of 10! Nevertheless, some interesting observations can be made with the caveat of so small a study and, as always, additional questions raised.

The communication between residents and their patients was medically dominated and biomedical in focus. This should not be surprising as the majority of medical visits have been characterized in this way in the theoretical and empirical literature (Roter & Hall, 1992). The pattern of resident communication was similar to a "biomedically-expanded" model of exchange described in earlier studies (Roter et al., 1997). Interestingly, younger physicians, including 3rd-year residents, were found to use the biomedical patterns of communication more than experienced physicians.

What was surprising was how biomedically focused the attending physicians' contribution was to the dialogue. Although we could not find any descriptions in the literature of attending physicians' dialogue with residents, we thought that as mentors and teachers to less experienced physicians, attendings would model more collaborative patterns of communication by greater inclusion of inquiry and counseling in the psychosocial domain. What we found was that attending physicians were less verbally engaged in the more psychosocial visits. Most interesting was attendings' greater use of activating and partnering with residents who did not explore psychosocial issues with their patients. Our interpretation of this finding is that the attendings engaged in more probing of residents' opinions and thought processes in the biomedical domain.

We could think of several explanations for this finding. The more psychosocial visits may have been less medically complex and less demanding of attendings' attention. Other studies have found that psychosocial issues are less often explored with sicker patients (Hall, Roter, Milburn, & Daltroy, 1996). We explored the array of patient problems, as best we could determine, but could not find an obvious connection between problem complexity or severity and the extent of psychosocial or biomedical focus. It is possible that the visits were not more biomedically complicated, but that both residents and attendings felt more comfortable discussing biomedical rather than psychosocial issues in the presence of the patient, or that residents felt that consultations were more appropriate for biomedical problems. In a similar vein, attendings may have felt more comfortable jumping into the dialogue of the visit in the biomedical rather than psychosocial sphere because the problems are technical in nature and more easily and directly addressed, whereas social and psychological problems may be thought to be too complex for a short consultation.

For whatever the reason, it is a loss that attendings did not address the psychosocial contexts of patients' problems in this study. Both patient and physician are dissatisfied with narrowly biomedical patterns of communication. Indeed, physicians rated patients with whom they had narrow biomedical visits as poor historians who provide low-quality data and make poor use of physician time. Physicians also saw these exchanges as least likely to achieve their visit goals (Roter et al., 1997).

The supportive function of communication may be seen at the intersection of the patient's experience and the physician's expertise. Interviewing skills that go beyond the biomedical paradigm to address the patient's life context hold the key to personal, responsive, and fulfilling communication between patients and physicians (Engel, 1988; McWhinney, 1989; Mishler, 1984). These skills will continue to be the most meaningful training challenge to help nurture and develop the capacity of meaningful autonomy and sensitive and respectful medical care.

## REFERENCES

Bales, R. F. (1950). *Interaction process analysis.* Cambridge, MA: Addison-Wesley.

Ben-Sira, Z. (1976). The function of the professional's affective behavior in client satisfaction: A revised approach to social interaction theory. *Journal of Health and Social Behavior, 17,* 3–11.

Ben-Sira, Z. (1980). Affective and instrumental components in the physician–patient relationship: An additional dimension of interaction theory. *Journal of Health and Social Behavior, 21,* 170–181.

Cohen-Cole, S. (1991). *The medical interview: The three function approach.* St. Louis, MO: Mosby.

Crain, E. F., Mortimer, K. M., Bauman, L. J., Kercsmar, C., Weiss, K., Wissow, L. S., Mitchell, H., & Roter, D. (1999). Pediatric asthma care in the emergency department: Measuring the quality of history-taking and discharge planning. *Journal of Asthma, 36,* 129–138.

Davis, M. (1969). Variations in patients' compliance with doctors' advice: An empirical analysis of patterns of communication. *American Journal of Public Health, 58,* 274–288.

Emerson, R. M. (1976). Social exchange theory. *Annual Review of Public Health, 2,* 335–362.

Engel, G. L. (1988). How much longer must medicine's science be bound by a seventeenth century world view? In K. White (Ed.), *The task of medicine: Dialogue at Wickenburg* (pp. 113–136). Menlo Park, CA: Kaiser Foundation.

Ford, S., Fallowfield, L., & Lewis, S. (1996). Doctor–patient interactions in oncology. *Social Science and Medicine, 42,* 1511–1519.

Freire, P. (1983). *Education for critical consciousness.* New York: Continuum Press.

Gouldner, A. W. (1960). The norm of reciprocity: A preliminary statement. *American Sociological Review, 26,* 161–179.

Greenfield, S., Kaplan, S., & Ware, J. E. (1985). Expanding patient involvement in care. *Annals of Internal Medicine, 102,* 520–528.

Hall, J., Roter, D., & Katz, N. (1987). Task versus socioemotional behaviors in physicians. *Medical Care, 25,* 437–451.

Hall, J., Roter, D., & Katz, N. (1988). Correlates of provider behavior: A meta-analysis. *Medical Care, 26,* 657–675.

Hall, J. A., Roter, D. L., Milburn, M. A., & Daltroy, L. H.. (1996). Patients' health status as a predictor of physician and patient behavior in medical visits: A synthesis of four studies. *Medical Care, 34,* 1205–1218.

Hall, J., Roter, D., & Rand, C. (1981). Communication of affect between patients and physicians. *Journal Health & Social Behavior, 11,* 18–30.

Lazare, A., Putnam, S. M., & Lipkin, M. (1995). Three functions of the medical interview. In M. Lipkin, S. M. Putnam, & A. Lazare (Eds.), *The medical interview: Clinical care, education, and research* (pp. 3–19). New York: Springer-Verlag.

McWhinney, I. (1989). The need for a transformed clinical method. In M. Stewart & D. Roter (Eds.), *Communicating with medical patients* (pp. 25–40). Newbury Park, CA: Sage.

Mead, N., & Bower, P. (2000). Measuring patient-centeredness: A comparison of three observation-based instruments. *Patient Education and Counseling, 39,* 71–80.

Mishler, E. G. (1984). *The discourse of medicine: Dialectics of medical interviews.* Norwood, NJ: Ablex.

Parsons, T. (1951). *The social system.* Glencoe, IL: Free Press.

Roter, D. L. (1987). An exploration of health education's responsibility for a partnership model of client–provider relations. *Patient Education and Counseling, 9,* 25–31.

Roter, D. L. (1999). *Roter interaction analysis system (RIAS): Coding manual.* Unpublished manual, Department of Health Policy and Management, Johns Hopkins School of Public Health, Baltimore.

Roter, D. L. (2000a). The enduring and evolving nature of the patient–physician relationship. *Patient Education and Counseling, 39,* 5–15.

Roter, D. L. (2000b). The medical visit context of treatment decision-making and the therapeutic relationship. *Health Expectations, 3,* 17–25.

Roter, D., & Hall, J. (1989). Studies of doctor–patient interaction. *Annual Review of Public Health, 10,* 163–180.

Roter, D. L., & Hall, J. A. (1991). Health education theory: An application to the process of patient–provider communication. *Health Education Research Theory and Practice, 6,* 185–193.

Roter, D. L., & Hall, J. A. (1992). *Doctors talking to patients/patients talking to doctors: Improving communication in medical visits.* Westport, CT: Auburn.

Roter, D., Hall, J., & Katz, N. (1988). Patient–physician communication: A descriptive summary of the literature. *Patient Education and Counseling, 12,* 99–119.

Roter, D., Lipkin, M., Jr., & Korsgaard, A. (1991). Gender differences in patients' and physicians' communication during primary care medical visits. *Medical Care, 29,* 1083–1093.

Roter, D. L., Stewart, M., Putnam, S., Lipkin, M., Stiles, W., & Inui, T. (1997). Communication patterns of primary care physicians. *Journal of the American Medical Association, 270,* 350–355.

Tuckett, D., Boulton, M., Olson, C., & Williams, A. (1985). *Meetings between experts.* New York: Tavistock.

Wallerstein, N., & Bernstein, E. (1988). Empowerment education: Freire's ideas adapted to health education. *Health Education Quarterly, 15,* 379–394.

Wissow, L. S., Roter, D., Bauman, L. J., Crain, E., Kercsmar, C., Weiss, K., Mitchell, H., & Mohr, B. (1998). Patient provider communication during the emergency department care of children with asthma. *Medical Care, 36,* 1439–1450.

# APPENDIX:
## SUPPLEMENTAL BIBLIOGRPAHY OF ROTER
## INTERACTION ANALYSIS SYSTEM (RIAS) STUDIES

### RIAS Use in Evaluating Communication Skills

deNegri, B., DiPrete Brown, L., Hernandez, O., Rosenbaum, J., & Roter, D. (1997). *Improving interpersonal communication between health care providers and clients.* Quality Assurance Methodology Refinement Series, Center for Human Services.

Hall, J., & Roter, D. (1988). Physician's clinical knowledge and compliance consciousness: Predictors of performance with simulated patients. *Evaluation and the Health Professions, 11,* 306–317.

Levinson, W., & Roter, D. (1993). The effects of two continuing medical education programs on communication skills of practicing primary care physicians. *Journal of General Internal Medicine, 8,* 318–324.

Roter, D. L., Cole, K. A., Kern, D. E., Barker, L. R., & Grayson, M. (1990). An evaluation of residency training in interviewing skills and the psychosocial domain of medical practice. *Journal of General Internal Medicine, 5,* 347–454.

Roter, D., & Ewart, C. (1992). Emotional inhibition in essential hypertension: Obstacle to communication during medical visits? *Health Psychology, 11*, 163–169.

Roter, D., & Hall, J. (1987). Physician interviewing styles and medical information obtained from patients. *Journal of General Internal Medicine, 2*, 326–329.

Roter, D. L., Hall, J. A., Kern, D. E., Barker, L. R., Cole, K. A., & Roca, R. P. (1995). Improving physicians' interviewing skills and reducing patients' emotional distress: A randomized clinical trial. *Archives of Internal Medicine, 155*, 1877–1884.

Roter, D. L., Rosenbaum, J., deNegri, B., Renaud, D., DiPrete-Brown, L., & Hernandez, O. (1998). The effectiveness of a continuing medical education program in interpersonal communication skills on physician practice and patient satisfaction in Trinidad and Tobago. *Medical Education, 32*, 181–189.

Van der Pasch, M., & Verhaak, P. F. M. (1998). Communication in general practice: Recognition and treatment of mental illness. *Patient Education and Counseling, 33*, 97–112.

Wissow, L. S., Roter, D. L., & Wilson, M. E. H. (1994). Pediatrician interview style and mothers' disclosure of psychosocial issues. *Pediatrics, 93*, 289–295.

## RIAS Relationships to Outcomes

Bertakis, K. D., Roter, D. L., & Putnam, S. M. (1991). The relationship of physician medical interview style to patient satisfaction. *Journal of Family Practice, 32*, 175–181.

Rost, K. M., Roter, D., Bertakis, K., & Quill, T. (1990). Doctor–patient familiarity and patient recall of medication changes. *Family Medicine, 22*, 453–457.

Rost, K., Roter, D., Quill, T., & Bertakis, K. (1990). Capacity to remember prescription drug changes: Deficits associated with diabetes. *Diabetes Research and Clinical Practice, 10*, 183–187.

Roter, D. L. (1977). Patient participation in the patient–provider interaction: The effects of patient question asking on the quality of interaction, satisfaction, and compliance. *Health Education Monographs, 50*, 281–315.

Roter, D., Hall, J., & Katz, N. (1987). Relations between physicians' behaviors and patients' satisfaction, recall, and impressions: An analogue study. *Medical Care, 25*, 399–412.

Roter, D. L., Hall, J. A., Kern, D. E., Barker, L. R., Cole, K. A., & Roca, R. P. (1995). Improving physicians' interviewing skills and reducing patients' emotional distress: A randomized clinical trial. *Archives of Internal Medicine, 155*, 1877–1884.

Roter, D. L., Stewart, M., Putnam, S., Lipkin, M., Stiles, W., & Inui, T. (1997). Communication patterns of primary care physicians. *Journal of the American Medical Association, 270*, 350–355.

Wissow, L. S., Roter, D., Bauman, L. J., Crain, E., Kercsmar, C., Weiss, K., Mitchell, H., & Mohr, B. (1998). Patient–provider communication during the emergency department care of children with asthma. *Medical Care, 36*, 1439–1450.

## RIAS Relationships to Patient and Physician Sex

Hall, J. A., Irish, J. T., Roter, D. L., Ehrlich, C. M., & Miller, L. H. (1994a). Gender in medical encounters: An analysis of physician and patient communication in a primary care setting. *Health Psychology, 13*, 384–392.

Hall, J. A., Irish, J. T., Roter, D. L., Ehrlich, C. M., & Miller, L. H. (1994b). Satisfaction, gender, and communication in medical visits. *Medical Care, 32*, 1216–1231.

Hall, J. A., & Roter, D. L. (1995). Patient gender and communication with physicians: Results of a community-based study. *Women's Health: Research on Gender, Behavior, and Policy, 1*, 77–95.

Roter, D., Lipkin, M., Jr., & Korsgaard, A. (1991). Gender differences in patients' and physicians' communication during primary care medical visits. *Medical Care, 29*, 1083–1093.

## RIAS Applications Outside of Primary Care

Ford, S., Fallowfield, L., Hall, A., & Lewis, S. (1995). The influence of audiotapes on patient participation in the cancer consultation. *European Journal of Cancer, 31A,* 2264–2269.

Ford, S., Fallowfield, L., & Lewis, S. (1996). Doctor–patient interactions in oncology. *Social Science and Medicine, 42,* 1511–1519.

Hampson, S. E., McKay, H. G., & Glasgow, R. E. (1996). Patient–physician interactions in diabetes management: Consistencies and variation in the structure and content of two consultations. *Patient Education and Counseling, 29,* 49–58.

Levinson, W., Roter, D. L., Mullooly, J., Dull, V., & Frankel, R. (1997). Doctor–patient communication: A critical link to malpractice in surgeons and primary care physicians. *Journal of the American Medical Association, 277,* 553–559.

Roter, D. L., Geller, G., Bernhardt, B. A., Larson, S. M., & Doksum, T. (1999). Effects of obstetrician gender on communication and patient satisfaction. *Obstetrics and Gynecology, 93,* 635–640.

Roter, D. L., Knowles, N., Somerfield, M., & Baldwin, J. (1990). Routine communication in sexually transmitted disease clinics: An observational study. *American Journal of Public Health, 80,* 605–606.

Roter, D., Roter, H., & Feinstein, M. (1984). Podiatrist–patient interaction during routine podiatry visits. *Journal of the American Podiatry Association, 74,* 553–558.

Sondell, K., Sonderfeldt, B., & Palmqvist, S. (1998). A method for communication analysis in prosthodontics. *Acta Odontologica Scandinavica, 56,* 48–56.

Wissow, L. S., Roter, D., Bauman, L. J., Crain, E., Kercsmar, C., Weiss, K., Mitchell, H., & Mohr, B. (1998). Patient–provider communication during the emergency department care of children with asthma. *Medical Care, 36,* 1439–1450.

# The Use of a Verbal Response Mode Coding System in Determining Patient and Physician Roles in Medical Interviews

Ayesha Shaikh, Lynne M. Knobloch, and William B. Stiles

*Department of Psychology*
*Miami University*

According to classic descriptions by Parsons (1951, 1969), the physician's role in medical interviews is characterized by high status and control vis-à-vis the patient. These complementary roles are not static, however, but shift substantially as the interview proceeds from taking a medical history, to conducting a physical examination, to concluding the interview with explanations and treatment plans. That is, although such interviews may be highly scripted—following a normative pattern that is predictable across patients and occasions—they are also complex, requiring a sequence of different relations between the roles to complete the necessary tasks. We used a verbal response mode (VRM; Stiles, 1992) coding system to derive quantitative indexes of physician and patient roles in three segments of each of eight medical interviews. We then used the indexes to characterize some of the complexity of these encounters.

## SEGMENTS OF MEDICAL INTERVIEWS

As described in standard interviewing texts (e.g., Billings & Stoeckle, 1998), medical interviews are typically a structured sequence of at least three distinct segments—a medical history, a physical examination, and a conclusion. Each of these segments has different tasks and purposes; hence, the relationship between patient

Requests for reprints should be sent to William B. Stiles, Department of Psychology, Miami University, Oxford, OH 45056. E-mail: stileswb@muohio.edu

and physician is different, and the resulting communication between patient and physician is different, across the three segments.

Ideally, in the medical history segment, the patient describes his or her problem in an attempt to inform the physician about his or her condition. The physician directs the conversation by inquiring about the history of the problem and other relevant background data, and listens attentively while the patient shares information.

In the physical examination segment, the physician makes direct observations, performs tests, looks for signs, and elicits patient responses to diagnostic procedures. The patient's role is to cooperate with the physician's instructions. The physician and patient must listen attentively to each other—the patient to respond appropriately to the physician's instructions and the physician to learn from the patient's reactions to the physical examination. During the physical examination, the physician has social license to be far more controlling and presumptuous than he or she would in daily life. A physician who was highly acquiescent and deferent during the physical examination might be viewed by the patient as incompetent.

In the conclusion segment, the physician prescribes treatment; provides explanations; answers questions; and gives instructions for further tests, return visits, medication dosages, and so forth. The patient listens attentively to the physician, agrees to follow directions, and asks questions about explanations or instructions that he or she does not understand. Physicians may still be somewhat controlling and presumptuous, but a physician who extended the same high degree of control in the conclusion segment as in the examination (by giving instructions and prescriptions without explanation, for instance) would likely alienate the patient.

## ROLE DIMENSIONS MEASURED BY VRMS

The VRM taxonomy offers a method of examining communication and quantifying status and relational aspects of physician and patient roles based on an utterance-by-utterance classification of verbal behavior (Stiles, 1992). Utterance-level codes are combined to yield indexes of three bipolar role dimensions: attentiveness versus informativeness, directiveness versus acquiescence, and presumptuousness versus unassumingness. As shown in Table 1, each of the taxonomy's eight basic modes is considered as either attentive or informative, as either directive or acquiescent, and as either presumptuous or unassuming. Importantly, VRM coders do not rate global qualities such as attentiveness directly; instead, they decide whether each utterance is a disclosure, a question, or one of the other six categories.

*Attentiveness* refers to a speaker's attention to the other person. Technically, utterances that concern the other person's experience (questions, acknowledgments, interpretations, and reflections) are considered as attentive (Stiles, 1992). For example, when one asks a question of another, the topic of the utterance is information held by the other person. Likewise, when a person uses a reflection, he or she

TABLE 1
Taxonomy of Verbal Response Modes Cross-Classified by Role Dimensions

| Dimension | Presumptuous | Unassuming |
|---|---|---|
| *Attentive* | | |
| Directive | Interpretation | Question |
| | Form: Second person ("you"); verb implies an attribute or ability of the other; terms of evaluation | Form: Interrogative, with inverted subject–verb order or interrogative words |
| | Intent: Explains or labels the other; judgments or evaluations of other's experience or behavior | Intent: Requests information or guidance |
| Acquiescent | Reflection | Acknowledgment |
| | Form: Second person ("you"); verb implies internal experience or volitional action | Form: Nonlexical or contentless utterances; terms of address or salutation |
| | Intent: Puts other's experience into words; repetitions, restatements, clarifications | Intent: Conveys receipt of, or receptiveness to, other's communication; simple acceptance, salutations |
| *Informative* | | |
| Directive | Advisement | Disclosure |
| | Form: Imperative, or second person with verb of permission, prohibition, or obligation | Form: Declarative; first person singular ("I") or first person plural ("we") where other is not a referent |
| | Intent: Attempts to guide behavior; suggestions, commands, permission, prohibition | Intent: Reveals thoughts, feelings, wishes, perceptions, or intentions |
| Acquiescent | Confirmation | Edification |
| | Form: First person plural ("we") in which referent includes other | Form: Declarative; third person (e.g., "he," "she," "it") |
| | Intent: Compares speaker's experience with other's; agreement, disagreement, shared experience or belief | Intent: States objective information |

*Note.* Both the form and intent of each utterance are coded. For example, "Would you close the window?" is question form with advisement intent.

is being attentive by using an utterance that is concerned with the other person's experience. *Informative utterances* (disclosures, edifications, advisements, and confirmations), on the other hand, concern the speaker's own experience. For example, disclosures of thoughts, feelings, wishes, perceptions, or intentions concern the speaker's experience.

Theoretically, physicians should gather information about their patients primarily during the medical history and physical examination segments of the medical interview, so one would expect physicians to be highly attentive during these segments. During the conclusion segment, however, physicians should be prescribing treatments and providing explanations to patients. Thus, one would expect physicians to be more informative in the conclusion segment by speaking from their own knowledge and experience. Patients would be expected to demonstrate a reciprocal pattern in these segments by being highly informative during the history and exam and more attentive during the conclusion segment.

*Directiveness* refers to guiding the conversation. Technically, utterances that use the speaker's frame of reference or viewpoint (disclosures, questions, advisements, and interpretations) are considered as directive. For example, asking a question points the conversation in a direction determined by the speaker. *Acquiescent utterances* (edifications, acknowledgments, confirmations, and reflections) allow the other's viewpoint to determine the course of conversation. For example, a reflection, which puts the other person's experience into words, is aimed at capturing and restating the other person's viewpoint.

Theoretically, part of the physician's role during medical interviews is to dictate the content of the interaction, based on his or her medical expertise. Hence, one would expect the physician to be more directive than the patient in all segments of the interview. Conversely, patients would be expected to be more acquiescent than physicians in all interview segments.

In *presumptuous utterances* (advisements, interpretations, confirmations, and reflections), a speaker expressly presumes knowledge about the other person. For example, when one uses a reflection, one presumes to understand the other's experience. Similarly, when one uses an advisement (guiding another person's behavior), one presumes to know what the other should do. *Unassuming utterances* (disclosures, questions, edifications, and acknowledgments) make no such presumption. For example, a disclosure (e.g., revealing personal thoughts or feelings) need not presume knowledge of the other's experience. Socially, presumptuousness is associated with higher relative status or prestige, whereas unassumingness is associated with lower relative status (Stiles, 1992).

Theoretically, because physicians have greater expertise and higher relative status than patients do, they have social license to be presumptuous. Patients are in a more supplicant, lower status role and may be expected to be unassuming toward their physicians. Thus, in a medical interview, one would expect the physician to be more presumptuous than the patient in all segments of the interview (but particularly during the physical examination, when the patient must disrobe and submit to being examined).

This study used the VRM role dimensions (attentiveness–informativeness, directiveness–acquiescence, and presumptuousness–unassumingness) to measure and describe the systematically changing relationship between patient and physician across the segments of the interview. The foregoing theoretical expectations are consistent with previous VRM research (e.g., Stiles, Putnam, James, & Wolf,

1979), with the observation that medical interviews have remarkably stable communication structures across a wide variety of patients, diagnoses, and settings (Stiles, 1996), and with descriptions of the doctor–patient relationship derived from clinical experience, textbooks, and other studies.

## METHOD

The VRM taxonomy was applied to eight transcripts of videotaped patient–physician interactions, which ranged from approximately 20 to 50 min in length. These interactions were interviews conducted by medical residents during a patient's initial visit. The patients presented with a variety of physical complaints. During the course of most of the interviews, an attending physician consulted with the resident physician about the case. (See Thompson's introduction to this issue for a more complete description of the videotaped interactions.)

Ten videotaped interactions were transcribed completely by collaborators in this special issue. Two of the 10 interactions that were transcribed could not be VRM coded because a large proportion of the dialogue was inaudible or incomprehensible. For the purposes of this study, the portions of the interviews that involved the attending physician were not included.

### VRM Coding System

The VRM taxonomy (Stiles, 1992) is a general purpose classification of speech acts. It concerns what people do when they say something rather than the content of what they say. Each *utterance* (defined as a simple sentence; independent clause; nonrestrictive dependent clause; multiple predicate; or term of acknowledgment, evaluation, or address) in dyadic conversation is classified according to the following three principles: (a) whether its topic is information held by the speaker or by the other (source of experience), (b) whether it is expressed from the speaker's point of view or from a point of view shared with the other (frame of reference), and (c) whether the speaker uses knowledge only of his or her own experience and frame of reference or presumes knowledge of what the other's experience or frame of reference is or should be (presumption). These three forced choices place every utterance into one of eight mutually exclusive VRM categories (see Table 1).

Each utterance is coded twice, once for its grammatical form and once for its pragmatic intent, using the same eight categories for each. Thus, an utterance can be a mixed mode and have the form of one mode and the intent of another. For example, "I went to the emergency room last week" would be coded DE, which means disclosure form (first-person singular) and edification intent (transmits objective information). An utterance can also be classified as a pure mode, having the same form and intent. For example, "I have pain when I move my legs" would be coded DD, which means disclosure form (first-person singular) and disclosure intent (reveals subjective experience).

As shown in Table 1, each mode is cross-classified by the three bipolar role dimensions (attentiveness–informativeness, directiveness–acquiescence, and presumptuousness–unassumingness). Indexes of each dimension are calculated as the proportion of a speaker's coded utterances (excluding uncodable utterances) in the designated modes. The role dimension indexes are calculated from utterance-by-utterance coding and are not based on global impressions. For example, attentiveness is calculated as the proportion of a speaker's coded utterances that were coded as reflection, confirmation, acknowledgment, or question. The index of informativeness is simply 1 minus attentiveness (because every coded utterance is either attentive or informative; see Table 1). In this study, we averaged the indexes across form and intent.

## VRM Coding Procedure

Each of the eight transcripts was coded independently by two coders (this article's first two authors) who were doctoral students in clinical psychology. The coders were trained using a computer-based training program and coding manual (Stiles, 1992), and they discussed practice transcripts with the third author before beginning work on this study.

The two independent raters agreed in distinguishing 6,849 utterances (utterances distinguished by only one coder were excluded), and they agreed on the VRM form of 85% of these utterances and on the VRM intent of 81% of these utterances. Discrepancies between the two coders were discussed and resolved, and a final consensus code for each utterance was used for subsequent analyses.

Each interview was divided into three segments—the medical history, the physical examination, and the conclusion. In each case, this was easily judged from the content, which explicitly signaled the beginning and end of the physical examination (e.g., beginning with the physician asking the patient to move to the examination table and ending with the physician leaving the room to consult with the attending physician). In one of the eight interviews, the physician resumed the physical examination after having begun the conclusion segment; in this case, we combined the two physical examination subsegments and the two conclusion subsegments for subsequent analyses. The parts of the interviews in which the attending physician was present along with the resident physician (approximately 15% of the total discourse) were excluded, leaving 5,840 utterances on which subsequent analyses were conducted. We excluded these passages because of the added complexity of having more than one possible addressee for utterances. For example, physicians are likely to be far less presumptuous in addressing each other than in addressing patients.

## RESULTS

Table 2 presents the mean indexes of patient and physician role dimensions (averaged across form and intent) in each of the three interview segments. The significance of the differences between the two roles (physician vs. patient) and among the three segments (medical history vs. physical examination vs. conclusion) was tested using 2 × 3 within-dyads analyses of variance. (We report tests only once for each bipolar dimension because these were identical for the two poles.)

Because role dimensions are derived from VRM categories, any differences can be examined more closely by considering the percentages of constituent VRMs in each profile. The patients averaged 242.0 utterances in the medical history, 55.9 in the physical examination, and 23.4 in the conclusion, whereas the physicians averaged 253.5, 108.0, and 44.2 utterances, respectively.

### Attentiveness–Informativeness

As expected, physicians tended to be more attentive than patients (and patients more informative than physicians) in the medical history and physical examination segments, whereas both had nearly equal attentiveness and informativeness in the conclusion segment (see Table 2). This was shown by a statistically significant role by segment interaction, $F(2, 14) = 8.28, p = .004$, as well as a significant main effect of role, $F(1, 7) = 13.59, p = .008$. The main effect of segment did not reach statistical significance.

TABLE 2
Mean Values on Role Dimensions Averaged Across Form and Intent of Utterances

| | Segment of Medical Interview | | | | | |
| | Medical History | | Physical Exam | | Conclusion | |
| Role Dimension | Patient | Physician | Patient | Physician | Patient | Physician |
|---|---|---|---|---|---|---|
| Attentiveness | 0.27 | 0.77 | 0.39 | 0.57 | 0.51 | 0.45 |
| Informativeness | 0.73 | 0.23 | 0.61 | 0.43 | 0.49 | 0.55 |
| Directiveness | 0.33 | 0.54 | 0.37 | 0.68 | 0.35 | 0.62 |
| Acquiescence | 0.67 | 0.46 | 0.63 | 0.32 | 0.65 | 0.38 |
| Presumptuousness | 0.05 | 0.22 | 0.06 | 0.34 | 0.14 | 0.33 |
| Unassumingness | 0.95 | 0.78 | 0.94 | 0.66 | 0.86 | 0.67 |

Note. For clarity, we present means for both poles of each role dimension. Because each role dimension index is equal to 1 minus the complementary index, however, half of these are technically redundant.

Physicians' very high attentiveness during the medical history segment was achieved mostly through the use of pure questions (e.g., "Who's been taking care of you?"; 28.5%) and acknowledgments—both pure acknowledgments (e.g., "mm-hm," "yeah"; 14.4% ) and interpretation forms with acknowledgment intent (evaluative words such as "right" or "okay" used to acknowledge receipt of information rather than to evaluate the patient; 13.5%). Patients' high informativeness included all four possible combinations of disclosure and edification form and intent: pure disclosure (e.g., "I'd feel like the muscles were numb"; 10.9%), disclosure form and edification intent (e.g., "I've been doing a lot of physical therapy"; 17.8%), edification form and disclosure intent (e.g., "Everything else seems okay"; 6.0%), and pure edification (e.g., "They said it was a pinched nerve"; 17.1%). During the physical examination, physicians continued to use many pure questions (20.7%) and pure acknowledgments (5.6%); however, they were somewhat more informative than in the history segment, particularly in their use of advisements (e.g., "Relax for me"; 14.2%). Correspondingly, patients used the informative modes disclosure and edification in the examination (edification form and disclosure intent = 12.5%, pure disclosure = 10.9%, pure edification = 10.2%, disclosure form and edification intent = 9.4%), but their increased use of pure acknowledgments (14.6%, up from 8.5%) was largely responsible for their slightly greater attentiveness than in the history segment. During the conclusion segment, physicians' much greater informativeness, as compared with earlier segments, was comprised mostly of a mixture of pure disclosures (12.8%), pure edifications (11.0%), and pure advisements (10.7%). Patients' reciprocally greater attentiveness included mainly acknowledgments—pure (16.4%) or with interpretation form (15.8%).[1]

---

[1]After coding was completed, we realized that the coders (i.e., the first two authors) had overlooked the VRM distinction between interpretation form and acknowledgment intent and interpretation form and confirmation intent (see Table 1). In the conclusion segment, patients use evaluative words (e.g., *right, okay*) both to indicate receipt of information, for example:

Dr: Your diastolic pressure is a little high [pure edification].
Pt: Okay [interpretation form and acknowledgment intent].

and to agree to comply with instructions, for example:

Dr: Call me if you notice any side effects [pure advisement].
Pt: Okay [interpretation form and confirmation intent].

The distinction is subtle, and the coding decision must rely on contextual cues, but the interpersonal transaction is different. In the latter case (confirmation intent), the patient was both informative (conveying an intention, making a contract) and presumptuous (necessarily presuming to know what the doctor means to agree to comply), whereas in the former, the patient has merely been attentive and unassuming (e.g., the patient could say "okay" without presuming to understand what was meant). The impact of some of the patients' evaluative words in the conclusion segment being confirmation intent instead of acknowledgment intent would be to slightly weaken our finding that patients tended to become less informative and strengthen our finding that they tended to become more presumptuous in the conclusion segment, as compared with the other segments.

## Directiveness–Acquiescence

Physicians were more directive than patients (and patients were more acquiescent than physicians) throughout the interview, especially during the physical examination segment (see Table 2). This was shown by a statistically significant main effect of role, $F(1, 7) = 31.49, p = .001$. There was also a significant main effect of segment, $F(2, 14) = 3.94, p = .044$, which reflected a slight but consistent tendency for both participants to be most directive during the physical examination and least directive during the medical history. The role by segment interaction did not reach statistical significance.

The modes by which physicians were directive changed across segments, in keeping with the content. During the medical history segment physician directiveness involved mainly pure questions (e.g., "Did they take x-rays of your neck?"; 28.5%); during the physical examination, it included both pure questions (e.g., "Does that hurt?"; 20.7%) and pure advisements (e.g., "Push against my hand"; 14.2%); and during the conclusion, it included many pure disclosures (e.g., "I'm going to make a quick phone call"; 12.8%), as well as pure advisements (10.7%) and pure questions (10.3%). Patients' relative acquiescence involved mainly edification forms and intents in the history segment as they answered physicians' questions (disclosure form and edification intent = 17.8%; pure edification = 17.1%; acknowledgment form and edification intent = 13.9%; edification form and disclosure intent = 8.5%); in the examination and conclusion segments, it included many pure acknowledgments as well (14.6% and 16.4%, respectively), as patients complied with procedural instructions and received directions for treatment regimens.

## Presumptuousness–Unassumingness

Physicians were consistently more presumptuous than patients, who remained almost completely unassuming through most of the interview (see Table 2). This was shown by a very large and statistically significant main effect of role, $F(1, 7) = 77.70, p = .0001$. Modifying this major difference were smaller tendencies for physicians to be relatively more presumptuous in the physical exam and conclusion, whereas patients were less unassuming in the conclusion than in the other two segments. Thus, the physician–patient gap in presumptuousness was largest in the physical examination and smallest in the conclusion. This pattern was shown statistically by a significant main effect of segment, $F(2, 14) = 7.10, p = .007$, and a significant role by segment interaction, $F(2, 14) = 6.50, p = .010$.

Physicians' relatively high presumptuousness during the medical history segment was achieved primarily through their use of pure reflections (5.3%). In the physical examination and conclusion segments, physicians' presumptuousness was represented primarily by their greater use of pure advisements (14.2% and 10.7%, respectively). Patients avoided the four presumptuous modes almost entirely, except that in the conclusion some of their utterances were interpretation form and acknowledgment intent (e.g., "okay," "right"; 15.8%). Using these evaluative words to convey receipt of information from the physician was considered slightly more presumptuous, in a formal sense, than using contentless, acknowledgment forms (e.g., "yeah," "mm-hm"; see also footnote 1).

## DISCUSSION

During the medical history, the physicians were highly attentive, moderately directive, and relatively presumptuous, whereas the patients were highly informative, moderately acquiescent, and extremely unassuming. The reciprocal pattern of physician attentiveness and patient informativeness seemed clearly consistent with the purpose of taking a medical history—for the physician to gain an understanding of the patient's condition. The physicians' relatively greater directiveness and presumptuousness, which continued throughout the interviews, seemed consistent with their authoritative role and high relative status, which allowed them to control the interaction and take conversational liberties that would not be accorded social equals (e.g., asking numerous questions and issuing commands without offering reasons).

During the physical examination, the physicians continued to be highly attentive (although slightly less so), and they increased their directiveness and presumptuousness, whereas the patients remained informative, acquiescent, and unassuming. These changes seemed consistent with the continuing purpose of gathering information coupled with the physicians' need to direct patients through examination procedures that (a) patients would not know how to do without explicit directions and (b) would be considered inappropriately intrusive and familiar in most other social settings.

During the conclusion segment, the physicians were somewhat less attentive, though they remained as directive and presumptuous as in earlier segments, whereas the patients became somewhat less informative, remained similarly acquiescent, and became a little more presumptuous (though still much more unassuming than the physicians). The summary effect of these shifts was that the roles converged somewhat, though the differences in control and status still remained large. The two roles' essentially equal informativeness–attentiveness in the conclusion is consistent with a mutual exchange of information between patients and physicians, as the physicians continued to seek information but also gave information, such as diagnoses, treatment instructions, and explanations about the illness and treatment. Perhaps because it involves a negotiation about possible courses of action, the conclusion may be considered as a more complex interaction than the earlier segments.

These shifts in role behaviors across segments are not at all surprising from a clinical perspective. However, theorists and researchers who conceptualize the physician–patient relationship in global terms, without considering systematic changes in roles during the medical interview, may overlook a crucial aspect of the relationship. Methodologically, a failure to separately analyze the medical history, physical examination, and conclusion segments could result in very misleading representations. For example, aggregated profiles might make a physician appear to be exceptionally directive and presumptuous with patients whose condition required an unusually extended physical examination. Distinguishing among segments would clarify what was taking place.

VRM coding allows researchers to quantitatively examine complex role relationships based on a systematic utterance-by-utterance classification. The VRM taxonomy is a general purpose system, which has been used to compare medical interviews with other sorts of interactions (e.g., psychotherapy, classroom discussion, courtroom interrogations; see Stiles, 1992) as well as with other interesting descriptors of medical encounters (e.g., demographic or diagnostic characteristics, patient satisfaction, adherence to prescribed treatment regimens). As this study demonstrated, coded utterances can be systematically aggregated into role dimensions that offer the advantages of both a broad, interpersonal conceptualization (in terms of attentiveness, directiveness, and presumptuousness) and the possibility of unpacking these abstract dimensions into specific utterances by participants. The results are consistent with clinical experience and descriptions in standard texts on medical interviewing (Billings & Stoeckle, 1998) as well as with previous VRM research (see Stiles, 1992, 1996). Because the abstract dimensions can be unpacked into specific behaviors, the taxonomy can be useful in training physicians to conduct medical interviews (Putnam, Stiles, Jacob, & James, 1988).

The generality of these results is limited by its small sample size, although the convergence with previous results (e.g., Stiles et al., 1979) lends some confidence. The fact that the coders were also investigators raises the possibility that their expectations may have biased the results, although it should be kept in mind that any bias would have to be expressed in the classification of particular utterances into VRM categories.

## REFERENCES

Billings, J. A., & Stoeckle, J. D. (1998). *The clinical encounter: A guide to the medical interview and case presentation* (2nd ed.). St. Louis, MO: Mosby.

Parsons, T. (1951). *The social system.* New York: Free Press.

Parsons, T. (1969). Research with human subjects and the professional complex. *Daedalus, 98,* 325.

Putnam, S. M., Stiles, W. B., Jacob, M. C., & James, S. A. (1988). Teaching the medical interview: An intervention study. *Journal of General Internal Medicine, 3,* 38–47.

Stiles, W. B. (1992). *Describing talk: A taxonomy of verbal response modes.* Newbury Park, CA: Sage.

Stiles, W. B. (1996). Stability of the verbal exchange structure of medical consultations. *Psychology and Health, 11,* 773–786.

Stiles, W. B., Putnam, S. M., James, S. A., & Wolf, M. D. (1979). Dimensions of patient and physician roles in medical screening interviews. *Social Science & Medicine, 13A,* 335–341.

# Analyzing Patient Participation in Medical Encounters

Richard L. Street, Jr. and Bradford Millay

*Department of Speech Communication*
*Texas A&M University*

An essential component of the delivery of health care is the consultation between the patient and health care provider. Participation in the medical consultation is fundamentally a communicative event in which clinicians and patients use talk to exchange information, to share their expertise and points of view, to build a trusting relationship, and to make health-related decisions. A growing body of evidence indicates that patients who more actively participate in these encounters are more satisfied with their health care, receive more patient-centered care (e.g., information, support) from providers, are more committed to treatment regimens, have a stronger sense of control over health, and even experience better health following the visit than do more passive patients (for reviews, see Kaplan, Greenfield, & Ware, 1989; Roter & Hall, 1993; Street, 2001). Because patient involvement is an important part of the health care process, it is imperative that investigators analyze the phenomenon using reliable and valid measures that have a solid conceptual foundation.

In this article, we have three objectives. First, we describe the conceptual foundation and measurement strategies used in our approach to analyzing the communicative acts that constitute patient participation in medical encounters. Second, we apply our method to an analysis of nine videotaped recordings of physician–patient interactions. Two research questions (RQs) will be examined: (a) To what extent do patients ask questions, express concerns, and engage in assertive behavior in their interactions with physicians? and (b) Are patients more active communicators when their physicians use partnership building (e.g., soliciting the patient's opinion) and supportive talk (e.g., reassurance, encouragement)? Finally, we conclude with a discussion of challenges and prospects for

Requests for reprints should be sent to Richard L. Street, Jr., Department of Speech Communication, Texas A&M University, College Station, TX 77843–4234. E-mail: r-street@tamu.edu

developing more ecologically valid and efficient procedures for assessing patient participation in care.

## ANALYZING PATIENT PARTICIPATION
## IN MEDICAL ENCOUNTERS

### Conceptual Foundation

To participate in medical consultations, patients must be able to express their needs, concerns, beliefs about health, and expectations for care (Street, 2001). For our purposes, we define *patient participation* as the extent to which patients produce verbal responses that have the potential to significantly influence the content and structure of the interaction as well as the health care provider's beliefs and behaviors. Patient participation can be conceptualized both qualitatively with respect to the types of speech acts that interject the patient's perspective into the consultation and quantitatively with respect to the frequency with which these behaviors are produced. Verbal acts of participation might include asking questions, descriptions of health experiences, expressions of concern, giving opinions, making suggestions, stating preferences, to name a few (Kaplan et al., 1989; Roter & Hall, 1993; Street, 1991, 2001).

### Measurement Issues

The most popular approach for studying the patient's actual behavior in the consultation is to first produce a transcript based on an audiotape or videotape of the interaction. Second, the interactants' responses are then divided into discourse units (e.g., utterances) and placed into particular categories of verbal behavior (e.g., questions, opinions). Quantitative indexes of the various discourse categories are then computed and used in statistical models either as a dependent variable (e.g., to test the effectiveness of a patient activation intervention; see Greenfield, Kaplan, & Ware, 1985; Roter, 1977) or as a predictor of outcomes of interest (e.g., patient satisfaction, adherence, health improvement; see Ong, de Haes, Hoos, & Lammes, 1995; Roter & Hall, 1993; Street, 1992a).

Although behavioral indexes of communication avoid some of the perceptual biases of self-report measures, they do have limitations. For one thing, the transcription and coding of interactions is slow and labor intensive. An interaction of 1 hr may take 3 to 4 hr to transcribe and code. Second, behavioral coding schemes often are not sensitive to within category differences in the interactants' perceptions of the coded units (Street, 1992a). For example, a physician might be more concerned if a 67-year-old patient said, "I have chest pains," than if he said, "I have a stomach ache," although both utterances could be coded as information giving.

## A PRAGMATIC APPROACH TO THE STUDY
## OF PATIENT PARTICIPATION

Aware of the strengths and limitations of behavioral approaches to the study of communication in medical consultations, our research team has developed a manageable, reliable, and theoretically grounded approach to the analysis of patient participation in care, one that can be used for a variety of scientific, clinical, and educational purposes.

### Operational Definitions

In previous research (Street, 1991, 1992a, 1992b; Street, Voigt, Geyer, Manning, & Swanson, 1995), we have identified three forms of speech—asking questions, expressing concerns, and assertive utterances—that are essential and observable features of patient participation in medical encounters. These types of responses are important because of their potential to influence the course of the interaction, elicit resources from providers (e.g., information, patient-centered care), and contribute to improved postconsultation outcomes. Table 1 provides definitions for these features of patient participation as well as some examples.

A question is an utterance in interrogative form, the purpose of which is to solicit information or clarification (Beisecker & Beisecker, 1990; Roter, 1977). An

TABLE 1
Operational Definitions of Communicative Acts of Patient Participation

| Verbal Behavior | Definition | Examples[a] |
|---|---|---|
| Asking questions | Utterances in interrogative form intended to seek information and clarification | "What's my thyroid?" "Does smoking do that?" "Is there anything they can do?" |
| Expressions of concern | Utterances in which the patient expresses worry, anxiety, fear, anger, frustration, and other forms of negative affect or emotions | "It's very frustrating" "No, ... I just have a fear of the operation" "I'm even scared to play with my own granddaughter" |
| Assertive responses | Utterances in which the patient expresses his or her rights, beliefs, interests, and desires as in offering an opinion, stating preferences, making suggestions or recommendations, disagreeing, or interrupting | "Go ahead and do it" "I really don't want anybody to x-ray it." "I don't want to have to lie for it" |

[a]These examples were taken from the transcripts used in this study.

expression of concern is a statement in which the patient expresses worry, anxiety, fear, anger (Street, 1991, 1992b), or other forms of negative affect (Kaplan et al., 1989; Roter & Hall, 1993). An expression of concern may be marked vocally by tone of voice or linguistically by such words as *concern, worry, afraid, frustrated,* or *mad.* Finally, a patient is being assertive when he or she expresses his or her rights, beliefs, interests, and desires during the interaction (see, e.g., Infante & Rancer, 1995). In a medical consultation, a patient is being assertive when stating an opinion about health, expressing preferences for treatment, making suggestions or recommendations, introducing a new topic for discussion, or disagreeing with the clinician.

## Coding Methods

In general, patients talk less than do physicians (about 40% and 60%, respectively), and most of their communication is in the form of giving information in response to the physician's questions (Roter, Hall, & Katz, 1988). Questions, expressions of concern, and assertive responses each on average represent less than 10% of patient's utterances (Roter et al., 1988; Street, 1992b). Because verbal acts of patient participation occur with relative infrequency, the first step in the coding process is to have coders simply listen to an audiotape or videotape of the interaction. Each time the coder perceives that a particular behavior occurred (e.g., the patient asked a question or expressed an opinion), that portion of the dialogue is transcribed including several conversational turns before and after the identified event. The next step is to divide the segment of discourse into utterances for coding. *Utterances* are the oral analogues of a simple sentence and may be in the form of a complete sentence, independent clause, nonrestrictive dependent clause, multiple predicate, or evaluation (Stiles, 1992). The coder then listens to that part of the tape again, follows the transcript, and places the utterances into mutually exclusive categories of verbal behavior (i.e., questions, expressions of concern, assertive utterances).

Although this sounds simple enough, there are factors that complicate our coding method. First, an utterance conceivably could fall into more than one category. Suppose a patient says, "Why did I get this disease?" In a normal tone of voice, this would be a question; in an emotional tone, this would be an expression of concern. Coders are instructed to code the act as he or she interpreted its primary function within the context of the discourse. Second, we have found that coding some types of assertive utterances is sometimes problematic. Expressing disagreement, interrupting, making a recommendation, stating preferences, and issuing directives are assertive acts that are relatively easy to identify. However, suppose a patient says, "I have borderline diabetes" or "I am a functional alcoholic." Are these simply observations about the patient's health status, or are they opinions emerging from the patient's personal beliefs about health? In our coding system, we generally take a conservative approach when patients express their views about health. These statements are considered assertive utterances only if (a) coders perceive them as an attempt by the patient to interject his or her beliefs into the interaction, and (b) the clinician explicitly accepts, challenges, or discusses this belief.

## Data Analysis

Because our samples of discourse usually are naturally occurring (and not the product of experimental manipulation), we generally rely on correlational and regression analyses to examine factors affecting and outcomes associated with patient participation in medical encounters. We do, however, try to control for confounding influences either by using a statistic, such as the semipartial correlation, which identifies unique variation shared between two variables (see, e.g., Street, 1991, 1992b) or by using regression procedures that first remove known influences on dependent variables prior to entering predictors of interest into the model (see, e.g., Street et al., 1993; Street & Voigt, 1997; Street, Voigt, et al., 1995).

Finally, a comment should be made about our choice to use frequencies of behaviors and not proportions (i.e., ratio of a particular behavior to the total number of behaviors produced by the interactant) as an index of patient participation. Although frequency and proportion data tend to be highly correlated, the argument could be made that frequency data are confounded by the length of the interaction, whereas proportion data are not. However, this claim ignores the fact that the discourse of medical consultations is mutually constructed by the interactants and that longer interactions will occur primarily because the participants choose to make more conversational contributions. Furthermore, our research indicates that frequencies of patients' and clinicians' verbal behaviors are generally more predictive of outcomes and are better predicted by theoretically meaningful variables (e.g., the patient's age and education, the physician's use of partnership building) than are behaviors coded as proportions (Street, 1992a).

## AN ILLUSTRATION

### RQs

As have the other authors in this special issue, we applied our coding system to the analysis of nine physician–patient consultations that were recorded on videotape. Although this is a small sample, we can address two important research questions.

RQ1: To what extent do patients in this sample ask questions, express conerns, and engage in assertive behavior during their interactions with physicians?

RQ2:  Are patients more likely to participate in these consultations when their physicians use partnership building and supportive talk?

As mentioned earlier, patient involvement in medical consultations can improve the quality of care patients receive and contribute to better health outcomes. Thus, assessing the degree to which patients participate in their interactions with physicians and identifying factors affecting their communicative activity are issues of considerable importance to both researchers and clinicians. In previous research, patient participation has been linked to (a) the patient's personal characteristics (e.g., age, education, personality; Beisecker & Beisecker, 1990; Street, 1992b, Street, Voigt, et al., 1995), (b) patient "activation" interventions designed to help patients become more involved in care (Greenfield et al., 1985; Rost, Flavin, Cole, & McGill, 1991), and (c) the health care provider's communicative style (Street et al., 1993; Street, Voigt, et al., 1995; Wissow, Roter, & Wilson, 1994). In this analysis, we examine patient participation in relation to the physicians' use of two types of patient-centered communication, partnership building and supportive talk.

*Partnership building* refers to communicative acts that encourage patients to discuss their opinions, express feelings, ask questions, and participate in decision making (Roter & Hall, 1993; Street, 1992a, 1992b). Partnership building also occurs when the clinician explicitly agrees with or affirms the patient's opinion, belief, or request. *Supportive talk* includes statements of reassurance, support, empathy, and other verbal displays of interpersonal sensitivity (Ong et al., 1995; Roter & Hall, 1993; Street, 1991). These verbal behaviors facilitate patient participation because they encourage and legitimize expression of the patient's views, needs, and concerns. Furthermore, conversational norms create expectations that the interactants' utterances be topically connected and that certain speech acts (e.g., answers) follow others (e.g., questions; Cappella, 1994; Sacks, Schegloff, & Jefferson, 1974). Thus, if asked by the physician, a patient is likely to state his or her preferences for treatment because the physician has provided an opportunity to discuss these issues and because the patient may feel obligated to share his or her views in light of the physician's request.

## Method

Nine videotaped physician–patient interactions were provided to the authors by the editors of this special issue of *Health Communication*. The patients were ethnically diverse (White, African American, and Hispanic) and balanced between men ($n = 5$) and women ($n = 4$). Four of the nine physicians were women. Transcripts of these interactions were prepared for coding purposes. Two trained coders, unfamiliar with the research questions, independently watched the videotapes while following the transcripts. As described in our earlier explanation of coding methods, the coders looked for and categorized utterances in which the patient asked questions, expressed concerns, and displayed assertiveness and utterances in which the physician used partnership building and supportive talk.

## Results

Table 2 presents the means, standard deviations, and ranges of physician and patient responses of interest. The first research question asked the degree to which patients participated in these interactions. Consistent with other research (Roter et al., 1988; Street, 1992b), patients varied considerably in their degree of participation, as some rarely asked questions, expressed concerns, and were assertive, whereas others were more expressive. Collectively, however, these acts of patient participation averaged less than 7% of the total utterances for patients. Also, as revealed in Table 2, physicians only occasionally used partnership building and supportive talk. These averaged less than 2% of the physicians' total utterances.

Other research similarly has shown that these types of verbal behaviors represent a small fraction of the talk of medical encounters (Roter et al., 1988; Street, 1992b). However, even by these norms, this sample of patients and physicians produced relatively few of the behaviors of interest. These responses may have occurred infrequently because, compared to patients in other studies, this small sample may have had less formal education, more ethnic diversity, and more physical ailments as primary complaints, variables that are generally associated with lower rates of patient participation and less patient-centered behavior (espe-

TABLE 2
Descriptive Statistics of Patient and Physician Responses

| Behavior | $M^a$ | SD | Range | % of Utterances[b] | Cohen's κ |
|---|---|---|---|---|---|
| Patients' participation | | | | | |
| Asking questions | 4.22 | 3.99 | 0–10 | 2.0 | .93 |
| Expressions of concern | 2.67 | 2.91 | 0–7 | 1.2 | .85 |
| Verbally assertive responses | 8.56 | 5.11 | 1–16 | 3.8 | .80 |
| Total active participation responses | 15.44 | 10.76 | 3–30 | 6.9 | .83 |
| Physicians' patient-centered responses | | | | | |
| Partnership building | 2.44 | 1.56 | 0–5 | 0.7 | .82 |
| Supportive talk | 2.78 | 2.43 | 0–7 | 0.8 | .85 |
| Total patient-centered responses | 5.22 | 3.08 | 1–11 | 1.5 | .81 |

[a]Mean scores represent the average frequency of the behavior for each interaction. [b]The percentages refer to the proportion of utterances of this type relative to the total number of utterances produced by that interactant. The mean number of patient and physician utterances per interaction was 233 and 348, respectively.

cially partnership building) by physicians (Kaplan, Gandek, Greenfield, Rogers, & Ware, 1995; Street, 1991, 1992b).

The second research question asked whether patients were more active participants the more their physicians used patient-centered responses. Because of the small number of interactions ($N = 9$) and the relative infrequency with which acts of interest occurred, the statistical relations between physicians' and patients' communication behaviors will be unstable. Nevertheless, these correlations were in the predicted direction, and several reached statistical significance (see Table 3). As expected, those doctors who used patient-centered responses in turn had patients who were more assertive, more freely expressed their concerns, and asked more questions. Moreover, the relation between patient-centered behavior and patient participation was sometimes bidirectional. That is, the patient's acts of participation appeared to encourage the physician to be more patient centered. The examples following, which were taken from these consultations, show how patient-centered responses can be both a stimulus for and response to acts of patient participation.

*Example 1:*
   Doctor:  Would you feel better if you had some support for your neck to wear once in a while? [partnership building]
   Patient:  What do you mean by that?
   Doctor:  Wear a collar?
   Patient:  On no ... not really. I feel uncomfortable with them on [assertive talk].

*Example 2:*
   Patient:  (I can) walk around, maybe you know, do a little housework. I do have my 8-year-old granddaughter that I have to take care of.
   Doctor:  Gosh, it seems awfully frustrating [supportive talk].

TABLE 3
Correlations Among Patient Participation Behaviors
and Physicians' Patient-Centered Responses

| | *Physicians' Patient-Centered Responses* | | |
| *Patient Participation Behaviors* | *Partnership Building* | *Supportive Talk* | *Total Patient-Centered Responses* |
| --- | --- | --- | --- |
| Asking questions | .72** | .25 | .71** |
| Assertive utterances | .70** | .27 | .64* |
| Expressing concern | .65** | .61* | .81** |
| Total patient participation behaviors | .76** | .41 | .78** |

*$p < .10$. **$p < .05$.

Patient:  I'm even scared to play with my own granddaughter ... scared I might hurt myself again [expression of concern].

*Example 3:*
Patient:  If you guys want me to keep coming for this, I will. But I do want to keep my doctor [assertive talk].

Doctor:  Yah, I think the important thing is to have a regular doctor that you consider your regular physician. I think that's very important [partnership building].

These examples highlight the prospect that the patient's efforts to participate in the consultation coupled with the physician's facilitation of this involvement can create a "cycle" of collaboration and rapport that ultimately leads to more patient-focused care and medical decisions that are better adapted to the patient's unique needs (Levenstein et al., 1989; Street, 2001).

Of course, there will be negative cases such as when the physician's partnership building fails to elicit greater patient involvement.

*Example 4:*
Doctor:  OK, do you have any questions or anything?
Patient:  No.

In other situations, the physician may be unresponsive or inattentive to the patient's question, concern, or preferences. In the example below, the patient persists in restating his opinion about eligibility for a disability assistance program until the physician finally responds.

*Example 5:*
Patient:  Cos, you know, I am, you know, partially disabled. Now I feel like I shouldn't have to lie for it (to get on SFI). What hurts me, you know, there's other people out there, you know, dope addicts ... alcoholics ... and, you know, people just acting like that [assertive talk].

Doctor:  Mmm.
Patient:  I don't feel like I have to lie for it [assertive talk].
Doctor:  Hmm.
Patient:  And I have to ... you know ... lie for it? Which I don't feel like I have to do [assertive talk].
Doctor:  What have they told you?

In summary, the evidence presented here suggests that physicians' use of partnership building and supportive talk does facilitate patient participation in medical consultations. Some clinicians might argue that greater patient involvement can be a problem because it takes up time in an already time-constrained visit. However, this is not necessarily the case, especially if providers feel less of a need to dominate the conversation as patients choose to talk more (see, e.g., Kaplan et al., 1989). Experienced and trained clinicians often need only a few minutes to listen to and satisfactorily discuss issues of concern to a patient (Branch & Malik, 1993), an amount of time that takes up only 5% to 20% of the consultation time available (Smith & Hoppe, 1991).

## CONCLUSIONS

In this article, we described the conceptual foundation and coding procedures for our method of investigating communicative behaviors underlying patient participation in medical encounters. Our approach is manageable and should be of value to researchers and clinicians interested in understanding and improving ways in which patients can participate effectively in the health care process. The limitations of our own and others' methods of studying provider–patient discourse highlight the need to develop even more valid and efficient measurement systems. Toward this end we see two important challenges, improving the interpretive reality of the coding system and developing more efficient coding methods.

### Improving Interpretive Reality

As mentioned earlier, verbal behaviors categorized as a particular type of speech act (e.g., giving information) may vary greatly in their perceptual salience to the interactants. A patient will respond very differently to "you have a cold" than to "you have cancer," although both utterances would likely be categorized as information giving. In a recent study, Street (1992a) explored the relation between perceptual and behavioral measures of communication and found that a quantitative index of physicians' information giving was not predictive of patients' perceptions of the doctors' informativeness. However, the same study did find that physicians who used fewer controlling and directive behaviors and who displayed more patient-centered responses were perceived by patients as more interpersonally sensitive and more actively engaged in partnership building.

Why would some behaviors be more closely linked to patients' perceptions than others would? One possibility deals with frequency of occurrence. Significantly more of the physician's time is devoted to giving information and asking questions than to partnership building and supportive talk (Roter et al., 1988). Thus, patient-centered responses may have high salience for patients because they are valued and relatively rare. Patients may be more discriminating with information giving because these responses occur more often and will vary in their perceived relevance (i.e., importance, novelty, clarity) to what the patient needs or already knows.

However, recognizing that a behavior of interest is a scarce but valued commodity does not address the overarching issue of how to converge behavioral categories with interactants' interpretations of the behavior. Several strategies may help this effort. First, investigators could adopt a "multiple measures" approach to analyzing communication by using both behavioral and perceptual measures (see, e.g., Street, 1992a, 1993, 1997; Street & Voigt, 1997; Street, Voigt, et al., 1995). A related approach is to combine qualitative and quantitative methods of analysis as we have done in this article (see also Roter & Frankel, 1992; Street, Gold, & McDowell, 1995). Quantitative analyses of verbal behavior allow researchers to discover the relation of discourse variables to each other and to outcomes of interest for an entire data set. On the other hand, quantitative measures are generally inadequate for capturing the underlying themes of discourse and the context in which they occur (Waitzkin, 1990). In this regard, qualitative methods (e.g., interpretive and critical analyses) may be very useful in understanding the rich complexities of the content and structure of discourse.

Finally, researchers could consider using stimulated recall, a methodological technique that requires the participants to review a recording of their consultation. As they listen or watch the recording, each interactant makes note of what he or she perceived as the significant events in the interaction. A major advantage of stimulated recall is that, rather than focusing on all of the behaviors exhibited during the exchange, the provider, patient, and (perhaps) coder can focus on the most notable behaviors that led to the most significant perceptions and outcomes. In this way, stimulated recall connects actual behavior to perceptual salience (cf. Frankel & Beckman, 1982).

## Improving the Efficiency of Coding Discourse

As just mentioned, the coding of verbal behaviors can be a laborious and time-consuming activity. If more investigators are to undertake the task of analyzing large samples of physician–patient discourse, efforts must be taken to streamline methods of observation and analysis. Several possibilities have potential in this regard. First, researchers can employ sampling procedures in which only a subset of the interactions are transcribed and coded. For example, researchers might analyze every 3rd min of the interaction, the first and last 5 min of the interaction, or the first 10 min of talk. By so doing, investigators are assuming that the distribution of talk in the segments of the interactions studied will be comparable to the pattern of talk for the entire interaction, an assumption that can be verified empirically.

Second, improvements in computing technology soon may help researchers reliably generate quantitative indexes of a wide variety of discourse features based on key words, forms of speech, and even paralinguistic cues. Currently available are programs that scan text to compute measures of content and style (see, e.g., Hart, 1984). These programs only partially reduce the need for human labor because a transcript of the interaction is needed as input into these programs. However, with new developments in voice recognition technology, we one day may be able to create indexes of verbal behavior based on audio signals alone. Of course, whether by machine or by human senses and interpretation, the coding of discourse will only be as good as the conceptual foundation of the coding system and the degree to which the measures generated and examples selected are connected to what interactants perceive and experience.

## REFERENCES

Beisecker, A. E., & Beisecker, T. D. (1990). Patient information-seeking behaviors when communicating with doctors. *Medical Care, 28,* 19–28.

Branch, W. T., & Malik, T. K. (1993). Using "windows of opportunity" in brief interviews to understand patients' concerns. *Journal of the American Medical Association, 269,* 1667–1668.

Cappella, J. N. (1994). The management of conversational interaction in adults and infants. In M. L. Knapp & G. R. Miller (Eds.), *Handbook of interpersonal communication* (2nd ed., pp. 380–418). Thousand Oaks, CA: Sage.

Frankel, R. M., & Beckman, H. B. (1982). Impact: An interaction-based method for preserving and analyzing clinical transactions. In L. S. Pettegrew, P. Arntson, D. Bush, & K. Zoppi (Eds.), *Explorations in provider and patient interaction* (pp. 71–86). Louisville, KY: Humana.

Greenfield, S., Kaplan, S., & Ware, J. E., Jr. (1985). Expanding patient involvement in care. *Annals of Internal Medicine, 102,* 520–528.

Hart, R. P. (1984). *Verbal style and the presidency: A computer-based analysis.* Orlando, FL: Academic.

Infante, D. A., & Rancer, A. S. (1995). Argumentativeness and verbal aggressiveness: A review of recent theory and research. In B. R. Burleson (Ed.), *Communication yearbook 19* (pp. 319–351). Thousand Oaks, CA: Sage.

Kaplan, S. H., Gandek, B., Greenfield, S., Rogers, W., & Ware, J. E. (1995) Patient and visit characteristics related to physician' participatory decision-making style. *Medical Care, 33,* 1176–1187.

Kaplan, S. H., Greenfield, S., & Ware, J. E., Jr. (1989) Assessing the effects of physician–patient interactions on the outcomes of chronic disease. *Medical Care, 27,* S110–S127.

Levenstein, J. H., Brown, J. B., Weston, W. W., Stewart, M., McCracken, E. C., & McWhinney, I. (1989). Patient-centered clinical interviewing. In M. Stewart & D. Roter (Eds.), *Communicating with medical patients* (pp. 107–120). Newbury Park, CA: Sage.

Ong, L. M. L., de Haes, C. J. M., Hoos, A. M., & Lammes, F. B. (1995). Doctor–patient communication: A review of the literature. *Social Science and Medicine, 40,* 903–918.

Rost, K. M., Flavin, K. S., Cole, K., & McGill, J. B. (1991). Change in metabolic control and functional status after hospitalization: Impact of a patient activation intervention in diabetic patients. *Diabetes Care, 14,* 881–889.

Roter, D. L. (1977). Patient participation in the patient–provider interaction: The effects of patient question asking on the quality of the interaction, satisfaction, and compliance. *Health Education Monographs, 5,* 281–315.

Roter, D. L., & Frankel, R. (1992) Quantitative and qualitative approaches to the evaluation of the medical dialogue. *Social Science and Medicine, 34,* 1097–1103.

Roter, D. L., & Hall, J. A. (1993). *Doctors talking to patients/patients talking to doctors.* Westport, CT: Auburn.

Roter, D. L., Hall, J. A., & Katz, N. R. (1988). Patient–physician communication: A descriptive summary of the literature. *Patient Education and Counseling, 12,* 99–119.

Sacks, H., Schegloff, E. A., & Jefferson, G. (1974). A simplest systematics for the organization of turn-taking for conversation. *Language, 50,* 696–735.

Smith, R. C., & Hoppe, R. B. (1991). The patient's story: Integrating the patient- and physician-centered approaches to interviewing. *Annals of Internal Medicine, 115,* 470–477.

Stiles, W. B. (1992). *Describing talk.* Newbury Park, CA: Sage.

Street, R. L., Jr. (1991). Information-giving in medical consultations: The influence of patients' communicative styles and personal characteristics. *Social Science and Medicine, 32,* 541–548.

Street, R. L., Jr. (1992a). Analyzing communication in medical consultations: Do behavioral measures correspond with patients' perceptions? *Medical Care, 30,* 976–988.

Street, R. L., Jr. (1992b). Communicative styles and adaptations in physician–parent consultations. *Social Science and Medicine, 34,* 1155–1163.

Street, R. L., Jr. (1993). Analyzing messages and their outcomes: Questionable assumptions, possible solutions. *Southern Communication Journal, 58,* 85–90.

Street, R. L., Jr. (1997). Methodological considerations when assessing communication skills. *Medical Encounter, 13,* 3–7.

Street, R. L., Jr. (2001). Active patients as powerful communicators: The communicative foundation of participation in care. In W. P. Robinson & H. Giles (Eds.), *The new handbook of language and social psychology* (pp. 541–560). Chichester, England: Wiley.

Street, R. L., Jr., Gold, W. R., & McDowell, T. (1995) Discussing quality of life in prenatal consultations. In G. H. Morris & R. Chenail (Eds.), *Talk of the clinic: Explorations in the analysis of medical and therapeutic discourse* (pp. 209–231). Hillsdale, NJ: Lawrence Erlbaum Associates, Inc.

Street, R. L., Jr., Piziak, V. K., Carpentier, W., Herzog, J., Hejl, J., Skinner, G., & McLelland, L. (1993). Provider–patient communication and metabolic control. *Diabetes Care, 16,* 714–721.

Street, R. L., Jr., & Voigt, B. (1997). Patient participation in deciding breast cancer treatment and subsequent quality of life. *Medical Decision-Making, 17,* 298–306.

Street, R. L., Jr., Voigt, B., Geyer, C., Manning, T., & Swanson, G. P. (1995) Increasing patient involvement in choosing treatment for early breast cancer. *Cancer, 76,* 2275–2285.

Waitzkin, H. (1990). On studying the discourse of medical encounters. *Medical Care, 28,* 473–488.

Wissow, L. S., Roter, D., & Wilson, M. E. H. (1994). Pediatrician interview style and mothers' disclosure of psychosocial issues. *Pediatrics, 93,* 289–295.

# Relational Control in Physician–Patient Encounters

Marlene M. von Friederichs-Fitzwater and John Gilgun
*Department of Communication Studies*
*California State University, Sacramento*

Effective communication between doctors and patients is a crucial determinant in optimum healthcare delivery (Bertakis, Roter, & Putnam, 1991; Inui & Carter, 1985; Stiles, 1989; Street, 1992). Increasing evidence indicates that effective physician–patient communication not only facilitates more accurate diagnosis and faster healing, but also improved patient understanding and comfort (Comstock, Hooper, Goodwin, & Goodwin, 1982; Husserl, 1984). However, it has only been since the mid-1960s that investigators began to study the interpersonal dynamics of physician–patient dyads with consistent methodological procedures (Roter & Hall, 1989; Roter, Hall, & Katz, 1988). Over the years, the research on physician–patient encounters has resulted in methodological diversity, a lack of theoretical cohesiveness or rational progression, and inconsistent, contradictory findings (Gilgun, 1997).

Part of the need for new and better methods to study physician–patient interactions has come out of changes in the healthcare model. Past research attention has been overwhelmingly focused on the interpersonal communication needs of providers, often overlooking the patients' needs (Kreps, 1988). Patient-centered medicine, also known as "reformed" or "transformed" medicine, has attempted to broaden the conventional biomedical approach (or disease-centered medicine) to include psychosocial issues of the patient and the family as well as the physician (Stewart & Weston, 1995). The patient-centered model not only includes the biomedical model, but also integrates all of the determinants of health in its method (Weston & Brown, 1995). This new model maximizes a collaborative partnership between doctors and patients (Roter & Hall, 1992) so that doctors may better understand their patients and their patients' needs and expectations. In this model, patients are encouraged to go through their own "agenda," not just the physicians' (Tate, 1983) and the patient is prompted to provide as much information as possible. Physicians need to allow pa-

---

Requests for reprints should be sent to Marlene M. von Friederichs-Fitzwater, Department of Communication Studies, California State University, Sacramento, 6000 J Street, Sacramento, CA 95819–6070. E-mail: fitzwaterm@csus.edu

tients to express ideas, expectations, fears, and feelings about their illness (von Friederichs-Fitzwater, Callahan, Flynn, & Williams, 1991). Physician behaviors deemed inappropriate include interrupting, discounting, or disregarding patient input or cutting off patient expression of ideas, expectations, feelings, or prompts (Levenstein et al., 1989; von Friederichs-Fitzwater et al., 1991).

The relational communication control method appears to provide a means for studying the physician–patient interaction as "relationship" and to broaden the focus of attention to include the patient as well as the physician. This method has been widely used to study informal dyads such as couples, marital pairs, families, and work pairs and only more recently to study formal dyads such as physician–patient and dentist–patient (Aneiros, 1993; Gilgun, 1997; O'Hair, 1989; von Friederichs-Fitzwater et al., 1991; Wigginton, 1995).

In 1989, O'Hair argued that health care systems could benefit from the direct application of relational communication theory. He stated that "negotiation of relational control in physician–patient relationships has important medical and legal implications" (p. 102). With the exception of one or two studies, more formal relationships had not been examined using relational communication methods until O'Hair's work. He chose to study the physician–patient relationship because it is a formal relationship in the sense that the participants meet for a limited time and for a specific purpose. In 1991, von Friederichs-Fitzwater et al. applied the method to examine the relationships of physicians caring for patients with terminal diagnoses and to compare the relational patterns of doctors and patients with less serious prognoses. McNeilis and Thompson (1995) examined the impact of relational control on patient compliance in dentist–patient interactions, and Wigginton (1995) used the method to examine family practice doctor–patient clinical encounters. Gilgun (1997) took a relational control approach to examine gender and control in family practice physician–patient dyads.

In the relational control method, the *transaction*—the exchange of paired sequential messages over time—becomes the basic unit of analysis. The relational coding scheme developed by Rogers and Farace (1975) was employed in the studies cited previously and in this study because it is appropriate for paired-sequential interactions and because it is more descriptive of relationships than other available methods. Rogers and Farace defined *relational control* in the theoretic concepts of symmetry, transitory, and complementarity. The relational communication model provides a method for examining the relational dimension of control (F. E. Millar & Rogers, 1987). The dimension of *control* is defined by F. E. Millar and Rogers as "establishing the right to define, direct, and delimit the actions of the dyad at the current moment" (p. 120).

Redundancy, dominance, and power are possible measures of control. *Redundancy* refers to the relational control efforts engaged in by the two people in a transaction. *Dominance* has to do with the degree of complementarity exchange of messages, whereas *power* focuses on the perceptions that people in a dyad have about the ability to influence and restrict behavior. A patient-centered model of healthcare suggests the need for shared control and a different way of communication for physicians and patients.

The relational control method is also founded on the relational control analysis work of Bateson (1958), Jackson (1959, 1965), Haley (1963), and Watzlawick, Beavin, and Jackson (1967), as well as the work on the operational level of Sluzki and Beavin (1965), Montgomery (1984), Spitzberg and Hecht (1984), Burgoon and Hale (1984), and Burgoon et al. (1987). The coding schema comes primarily from the work of Mark (1971) and Rogers and Farace (1975). Studies in control and communication by Northouse and Northouse (1987) and O'Hair (1989) also examined the methods that have been used to assess control in communication.

According to Ruesch and Bateson (1951), every message has two levels of meaning: (a) a report or control aspect that conveys information, and (b) a command or relational aspect, which defines the nature of the relationship between the two people. Two principal types of transactions have been defined on the basis of relational control: *symmetry,* which refers to the interchange of equivalent control messages, and *complementarity,* which refers to the interchange of maximally dissimilar control messages. Sluzki and Beavin (1965) defined *symmetrical interaction* as "equality and the minimization of difference" and complementary interaction as "maximization of difference." There are three basic types of symmetry: *competitive,* characterized by escalation for control; *neutralized,* characterized by mutual respect and by not taking a stand on the issue of control; and *submissive,* characterized by mutual coalescence and surrender (Fitzpatrick, 1988). Whether a transaction is symmetrical or complementary, both people in the dyad must participate in the definition of the relationship. Mark (1971) operationalized the concepts of symmetry and complementarity by developing a 3-digit code to designate each message. Rogers and Farace (1975) developed a transactional level coding system that focuses on message sequences, on indexing relational control, and on mapping transactional patterns as they unfold over time. F. E. Millar and Rogers (1987) further developed the propositions on relational communication by defining three relational dimensions (control, trust, and intimacy) and creating a model that clarified the behaviors intrinsic to the study of relationships. O'Hair (1989) linked the three relational dimensions to physician–patient relationships and argued for increased relational communication analysis in the healthcare context.

## METHOD

### Physician–Patient Interactions

For the purposes of this study, 10 physician–patient interactions were videotaped and transcribed for coding and analysis. The interactions were first time visits by patients in a family practice clinic in an urban teaching medical center. The relational control analysis focused on message sequences. A *message* was defined as each verbal intervention by participants in an ongoing dialogue. Each message was treated as both a response to the preceding message and a stimulus for the message that followed.

## Coding

A 3-digit code was assigned to each individual's utterance. The 1st digit represented the speaker (1 = doctor, 2 = patient), the 2nd digit indicated the format of the message, and the 3rd digit identified the response mode of the message (see Appendix A for message coding).

The 2nd digit, message format, requires fairly simple coding and "involves very little inference on the part of the coder" (Rogers & Farace, 1975, p. 229). The categories (assertion, question, talk-over, noncomplete, and other) required little interpretation. The 3rd digit, the response mode of the message, was coded using the definitions of the categories developed by Rogers and Farace (1975, pp. 229–230).

The 3-digit codes were then translated into control codes. The three types of control directions, as defined by Rogers and Farace (1975) are (a) one up ($\uparrow$), which indicates a movement toward gaining control of the interaction (e.g., orders, topic changes, instructions, etc.); (b) one down ($\downarrow$), which indicates a movement toward allowing, seeking, or accepting control of the interaction, such as support responses; and (c) one across ($\rightarrow$), which indicates a movement toward neutralizing control of the interaction (see Figure 1).

The control directions of the two speakers are then paired based on sequential responses. For example, a pair of responses from speakers with both assigned a

|  | Support | Nonsupport | Extension | Answer | Instruction | Other | Disconfirmation | Topic Change | Termination | Other |
|---|---|---|---|---|---|---|---|---|---|---|
| 1 = Assertion | $\downarrow$ | $\uparrow$ | $\rightarrow$ | $\uparrow$ | $\uparrow$ | $\uparrow$ | $\uparrow$ | $\uparrow$ | $\uparrow$ | $\rightarrow$ |
| 2 = Question | $\downarrow$ | $\uparrow$ | $\downarrow$ | $\uparrow$ | $\uparrow$ | $\uparrow$ | $\uparrow$ | $\uparrow$ | $\uparrow$ | $\rightarrow$ |
| 3 = Talk-Over | $\downarrow$ | $\uparrow$ | $\uparrow$ | $\uparrow$ | $\uparrow$ | $\uparrow$ | $\uparrow$ | $\uparrow$ | $\uparrow$ | $\rightarrow$ |
| 4 = Noncomplete | $\downarrow$ | $\uparrow$ | $\rightarrow$ | $\uparrow$ | $\uparrow$ | $\uparrow$ | $\uparrow$ | $\uparrow$ | $\rightarrow$ | $\rightarrow$ |
| 5 = Other | $\downarrow$ | $\uparrow$ | $\rightarrow$ | $\uparrow$ | $\uparrow$ | $\uparrow$ | $\uparrow$ | $\uparrow$ | $\uparrow$ | $\rightarrow$ |

FIGURE 1    Transaction control types.

| Control Direction of Speaker A's Message | Control Direction of Speaker B's Message | | |
|---|---|---|---|
| One-up | 1. ↑↑<br>Competitive Symmetry | 4. ↑↓<br>Complementarity | 7. ↑→<br>Transition |
| One-down | 2. ↓↑<br>Complementarity | 5. ↓↓<br>Submissive Symmetry | 8. ↓→<br>Transition |
| One-across | 3. →↑<br>Transition | 6. →↓<br>Transition | 9. →→<br>Neutralized |

FIGURE 2    Nine control configurations.

one-up code is described as *competitive symmetry* (↑↑), indicating that both speakers are competing for control of the interaction. A pair of one-down messages is called *submissive symmetry* (↓↓), with both speakers allowing control of the interaction. A pair of one-across messages is defined as *neutralized symmetry* (→→), meaning that neither speaker is allowing or attempting control of the interaction. Complementarity messages are those pairs that are one up/one down or one down/one up, indicating that if one speaker seeks control of the interaction, the other speaker yields, or if one speaker yields control of the interaction, the other speaker will seek control. Rogers and Farace (1975) further defined message pairs that were one across as *transitory:* One up/one across (↑→) and one across/one up (→↑) pairs are *transitory dominant; transitory submissive* are those pairs that are one down/one across (↓→) and one across/one down (→↓; see Figure 2).

## RESULTS

There were a total of 10 transcripts used in this study, with a total of 5,905 utterances. The analysis revealed that physicians produced a total of 2,955 utterances and patients produced a total of 2,950 utterances. The difference in utterances between relational partners came from physicians' beginning and ending interactions and from physicians' utterances that elicited no response from the patient. Table 1 reports the frequency of each of the nine transaction control types for both physicians and patients.

The findings reported in Table 1 indicate that the predominant transaction mode was transitory submissive (one down, one across), accounting for 21% of all relational transactions. Patients attempted control almost as often as physicians (126 vs. 243 times) did, but physicians were 6 times more willing (618 vs. 100) to assume control of the transaction when such control was offered (one down, one up). However, when physicians were neutral, patients were more than 7 times as willing to as-

TABLE 1
Frequency of Transaction Control Types

| | Physician | | Patient | | Total | |
|---|---|---|---|---|---|---|
| Control Type | No. | % | No. | % | No. | % |
| Up up | 243 | 4.1 | 126 | 2.1 | 365 | 6.2 |
| Down down | 171 | 2.9 | 202 | 3.4 | 373 | 6.3 |
| Up down | 118 | 1.9 | 661 | 11.2 | 779 | 13.2 |
| Down up | 618 | 10.5 | 100 | 1.7 | 718 | 12.1 |
| Neutral down | 213 | 3.6 | 973 | 16.5 | 1,183 | 20.0 |
| Neutral up | 51 | 0.86 | 361 | 6.1 | 412 | 6.9 |
| Up neutral | 233 | 3.9 | 120 | 2.0 | 353 | 5.9 |
| Down neutral | 1,047 | 17.7 | 203 | 3.4 | 1,243 | 21.0 |
| Neutral neutral | 261 | 4.4 | 204 | 3.5 | 465 | 7.9 |
| Total | 2,955 | 50.0 | 2,950 | 50.0 | 5,905 | 100.0 |

Note.    Neutral = across.

sume control (51 vs. 361). Interestingly, though, when physicians were assuming control, patients largely responded with one-down messages (118 vs. 661), indicating a willingness on the part of patients to assume control if physicians are neutral, but an unwillingness to wrest control when physicians give one-up messages. Table 1 also indicates that the second dominant transaction control type for the transactions was transitory submissive (one across, one down), accounting for 20% of the exchanges. Thus, over 40% of the relational transactions were symmetrical.

Table 2 reports the frequencies of the 10 relational categories for physicians and patients. Support is the most frequent relational category used by both patients and physicians, accounting for 32.7% ($n = 1,932$) messages. Physicians gave considerably more support than patients (1,516 vs. 416) did. Although the numbers were small, patients gave more nonsupport messages than physicians (14 vs. 2) did. Patients answered more questions (788 vs. 47) than physicians did, physicians gave more instructions (220 vs. 1) than patients did, and physicians changed the topic more than patients (149 vs. 14) did.

Table 3 reports the frequency of the six message format categories across all contexts. Overall, patients had slightly more assertions than physicians (1,544 vs.1,504) did, and assertions accounted for the largest ratio of messages for both patients (26%) and physicians (25.5%). The second category for physicians was questions (14%), and for patients was silence (14%). Patients were silent more than physicians (822 vs. 57) were, physicians asked more questions than patients (826 vs. 50) did, and physicians and patients talked over each other about equally (306 vs. 317).

Table 4 reports on the dimension of domineeringness as measured by the number of individual one-up messages divided by the total utterances and includes information on the gender of patients and physicians (see Appendix B for patient demographics). Domineeringness was clearly exhibited by the patients, particularly by male patients.

In contrast, dominance is measured by the ratio of one-up messages followed by one-down messages (dominance followed by submission). When physicians gave one-up messages, patients gave one-down responses in only 11.2% of the exchanges, indicating a lack of dominance. Likewise, when patients gave one-up messages, physicians responded with one-down messages in only 10.5% of the exchanges. When patients gave one-down messages, physicians responded with one-up messages in 1.9% of the exchanges; when physicians gave one-down message, patients responded with one-up messages in 1.7% of the exchanges. So although there was little evidence of dominance, what little dominance existed was

TABLE 2
Frequency of Relational Categories

| Category | Physician | | Patient | | Total | |
|---|---|---|---|---|---|---|
| | No. | % | No. | % | No. | % |
| Support | 1,516 | 25.7 | 416 | 7.1 | 1,932 | 32.7 |
| Nonsupport | 2 | 0 | 14 | 0.2 | 16 | 0.2 |
| Extension | 678 | 11.5 | 625 | 10.6 | 1,303 | 22.1 |
| Answer | 47 | 0.8 | 788 | 13.3 | 835 | 14.1 |
| Order | 6 | 0.1 | 0 | 0 | 6 | 0.1 |
| Instruction | 220 | 3.7 | 1 | 0 | 221 | 3.7 |
| Disconfirmation | 1 | 0 | 3 | 0 | 221 | 3.7 |
| Topic change | 149 | 2.5 | 14 | 0.2 | 163 | 2.8 |
| Termination | 4 | 0.1 | 3 | 0 | 7 | 0.1 |
| Other | 332 | 5.6 | 1,086 | 18.4 | 1,418 | 24.0 |
| Total | 2,955 | 50.0 | 2,950 | 50.0 | 5,905 | 100.0 |

TABLE 3
Frequency of Six Message Format Categories

| Category | Physician | | Patient | | Total | |
|---|---|---|---|---|---|---|
| | No. | % | No. | % | No. | % |
| Assertion | 1,504 | 25.5 | 1,544 | 26.0 | 3,048 | 52.0 |
| Question | 826 | 14.0 | 50 | 0.9 | 876 | 14.8 |
| Talk over | 306 | 5.2 | 317 | 5.4 | 623 | 10.5 |
| Noncomplete | 133 | 2.2 | 55 | 1.0 | 188 | 3.2 |
| Silence | 57 | 1.0 | 822 | 14.0 | 879 | 14.9 |
| Other | 129 | 2.2 | 162 | 2.7 | 291 | 5.0 |
| Totals | 2,955 | 50.0 | 2,950 | 50.0 | 5,905 | 100.0 |

TABLE 4
Domineeringness and Gender

| File No. | Physician | | Patient | |
|---|---|---|---|---|
| | % | Gender | % | Gender |
| 904 | 24 | Male | 31 | Female |
| 906 | 23 | Female | 31 | Female |
| 911 | 21 | Female | 26 | Female |
| 917 | 19 | Male | 28 | Male |
| 931 | 21 | Male | 29 | Female |
| 941 | 24 | Male | 29 | Female |
| 947 | 25 | Male | 32 | Female |
| 948 | 17 | Male | 41 | Male |
| 954 | 11 | Female | 32 | Male |
| 955 | 18 | Male | 33 | Male |

on the part of the physician. Domineeringness, however, was clearly exhibited by the patients.

## DISCUSSION

Both healthcare providers and patients depend on their communication to gather and provide information in healthcare situations (Maibach & Kreps, 1986), but we still do not know much about the complexities and subtleties of health communication as it is carried out in the medical encounter as we enter the next century. Analyzing doctor–patient encounters can provide information that will be helpful in better understanding this relationship and in providing high quality, patient-centered healthcare. In a managed care setting, there is also need to understand how to implement a patient-centered model within limited time constraints.

The physicians and patients analyzed in this study tended to concentrate their messages into only three of the nine possible relational categories: support, extension, and other. They also tended to use predominantly transitory symmetrical exchanges. It would first appear that symmetric relationships are the most desirable. After all, if the doctor and patient treat each other as equals, then struggles over dominance should disappear. Some researchers believe, however, that the dominance issue is more unsettled in a symmetrical relationship than in a complementary relationship. When people treat each other as equals, they may not be ignoring dominance, they may be in competition for it (Jackson, 1959). Paradoxically, "trying not to control" is an attempt to limit the other—by getting him or her to take the responsibility (Wilmot, 1980). By more closely examining the difference between dominance and domineeringness, it is possible to better understand the relationships of the doctors and patients in this study. A domineering statement is a one-up message whose purpose is conversational control. Only when it is responded to with a subsequent one-down response by the other is the result dominance (L. Millar, Rogers, & Millar, 1977). Dominance occurs when the other person cooperates, however implicitly, with our definition of the relationship at that particular time. Patients in this study clearly exhibited a tendency toward domineeringness, suggesting an unwillingness to give up control to the physicians.

Thus, although the findings in this study indicate a more equal relationship on the surface, on further examination, the interactions appear to be doctor centered or disease centered with a pattern of the doctor frequently changing the topic, asking more questions, and talking more than the patient. Patients, on the other hand, exhibit significantly greater domineeringness as they attempt to shift the power through relational control.

Power is a central concept to the understanding of how two individuals work out their relationship between themselves. Although power is vitally important in dyadic relationships, it is not synonymous with dominance. Exercising conversational control by interrupting, or making other one-up moves (dominance), is not the same as relational control. One can exercise relational control without dominating individuals' conversations. For example, in examining the transcripts of the physician–patient encounters included in this study, if the patient was silent and the physician responded to this submissiveness, the patient may be demonstrating relational power without exercising conversational dominance. It may be that these patients perceive the physicians to be higher in dominance, but are castigating their power use by making counter moves to more fully equalize it. There is also some evidence to suggest that if a relationship is parallel, that is if both complementary and symmetric definitions occur, the transactions are less rigid and less inclined to be pathological (Lederer & Jackson, 1968; F. E. Millar, 1973; Sluzki & Beavin, 1965; Watzlawick et al., 1967).

Because they exhibited a high degree of rigidity, the physician–patient relationships examined in this study would also appear to have agreement about individual roles. F. E. Millar (1973) developed a measure of the structure or rigidity of relational patterns by determining the extent to which a dyad concentrated its messages into a few relational categories rather than using all nine categories equally. He found that dyads with greater rigidity had more agreement and understanding about their relational satisfaction. He also found that dyads with greater rigidity tended to use symmetrical exchanges as the expression of their rigidity, rather than the other relational categories. West (1983) found that physician–patient talk is more constrained by utterance type and speaker identity than casual conversation. For example, not only do doctors ask the questions in the exchanges with patients, but also patients respond to them. In this study, patients answered 788 of the 826 (or 95%) questions asked by physicians. However, physicians also responded to the majority of patient questions (50 questions asked by patients; 47 answered by physicians). This differed from Korsch, Gozzi, and Francis's (1968) findings that indicated that patients' queries were commonly ignored. However, this study did agree with Korsch et al. with regard to frequent changes of subject by physicians. Physicians in this study changed the topic 149 times, whereas patients changed the topic only 14 times. Both physicians and patients tended to extend the topic equally (physicians 11.5% and patients 10.6% of the time), but the physicians controlled the topics.

Patients in this study seem willing to assume greater control and responsibility of their own health and healthcare, but appear reluctant to control the conversations they have with their physicians through more overt dominance. The encounters reported in this study were all first-time visits and this may have allowed the patients more opportunities to explore and establish boundaries in these developing relationships. Waitzkin (1991) pointed out several manifestations of social class and power differences that appear in patterns of language, silences, and disproportionate reciprocity. The patients in this study were also all low-income individuals receiving medical services from a clinic that serves those on government assistance and the "medically indigent." Patients of a lower social class may be reluctant to openly challenge physicians and choose, instead, to attempt to control the relationship. In terms of gender differences, male patients in this study were more domineering than the female patients regardless of the gender of the physician. Relational control method provides a way to examine the physician–patient relationship and seems suited to provide information about the process of communication in the healthcare setting.

Obviously, more research needs to be done to better understand the physician–patient relationship and to further define the communication strategies that will move the clinical encounter away from a doctor- or disease-centered model to a patient-centered model.

## ACKNOWLEDGMENTS

We wish to note that Rogers and Farace (1975) included neither a number 6 nor a category "instruction" in their numerical list of message code categories on page 228 of their article, even though the category "instruction" is defined on page 229. Von Friederichs-Fitzwater et al. (1991) modified the scheme by adding a number 5 "instruction" category.

## REFERENCES

Aneiros, M. (1993). *How patients and physicians talk in a medical consultation: A relational view.* Unpublished master's thesis, University of Wyoming, Laramie.
Bateson, G. (1958). *Naven* (2nd ed.). Stanford, CA: Stanford University Press.

Bertakis, K. D., Roter, D., & Putnam, S. M. (1991). The relationship of physician medical interview style to patient satisfaction. *Journal of Family Practice, 32*(2), 175–181.

Burgoon, J. K., & Hale, J. L. (1984). The fundamental topoi of relational communication. *Communication Monographs, 51,* 193–214.

Burgoon, J. K., Pfau, M., Parrott, R., Birk, R., Coker, R., & Burgoon, M. (1987, May). *Relational communication, satisfaction, compliance-gaining strategies, and compliance in communication between physicians and patients.* Paper presented at the International Communication Association Annual Conference, Montreal, Canada.

Comstock, L. M., Hooper, E. M., Goodwin, J. M., & Goodwin, J. S. (1982). Physician behaviors that correlate with patient satisfaction. *Journal of Medical Education, 57,* 105–112.

Fitzpatrick, M. A. (1988). *Between husbands and wives: Communication in marriage.* Newbury Park, CA: Sage.

Gilgun, J. (1997). *Gender and control in physician–patient dyads: A relational control approach.* Unpublished master's thesis, California State University, Sacramento.

Haley, J. (1963). Marriage therapy. *Archives of General Psychiatry, 8,* 213–224.

Husserl, F. (1984). Effective communication: A powerful risk management tool. *Western Journal of Medicine, 145,* 29–30.

Inui, T. S., & Carter, W. B. (1985). Problems and prospects for health services research on provider–patient communication. *Medical Care, 23,* 521–538.

Jackson, D. D. (1959). Family interaction, family homeostasis and some implications for conjoint family psychotherapy. In J. H. Masserman (Ed.), *Individual and family dynamics* (pp. 122–141). New York: Grune & Stratton.

Jackson, D. D. (1965). The study of family. *Family Process, 4,* 1–20.

Korsch, B. N., Gozzi, E. K., & Francis, V. (1968). Gaps in doctor–patient interaction and patient satisfaction. *Pediatrics, 42,* 855–870.

Kreps, G. L. (1988). Relational communication in health care. *Southern Communication Journal, 53,* 344–359.

Lederer, W. J., & Jackson, D. D. (1968). *Mirages of marriage.* New York: Norton.

Levenstein, J. H., Brown, J. B., Weston, W. W., Stewart, M., McCracken, E. C., & McWhinney, I. (1989). Patient-centered interviewing. In M. Stewart & D. Roter (Eds.), *Communicating with medical patients* (pp. 107–120). Newbury Park, CA: Sage.

Maibach, E., & Kreps, G. (1986, September). *Communicating with patients: Primary care physicians' perspectives on cancer prevention, screening, and education.* Paper presented at the International Conference on Doctor–Patient Communication, Centre for Studies in Family Medicine, University of Western Ontario, London, Canada.

Mark, R. (1971). Coding communication at the relationship level. *Journal of Communication, 21,* 221–232.

McNeilis, K. S., & Thompson, T. L. (1995). The impact of relational control on patient compliance in dentist/patient interactions. In G. L. Kreps & D. O'Hair (Eds.), *Communication and health outcomes* (pp. 57–72). Cresskill, NJ: Hampton.

Millar, F. E. (1973). *A transactional analysis of marital communication patterns: An exploratory study.* Unpublished doctoral dissertation, Michigan State University, Lansing.

Millar, F. E., & Rogers, L. E. (1987). Relational dimensions of interpersonal dynamics. In M. R. Roloff & G. R. Miller (Eds.), *Interpersonal process: New directions in communication research* (pp. 117–139). Newbury Park, CA: Sage.

Millar, L., Rogers, E., & Millar, F. E. (1977, November). *A transactional definition and measure of paper.* Paper presented to the Speech Communication Association Convention, Washington, DC.

Montgomery, B. M. (1984). Individual differences and relational interdependencies in social interaction. *Human Communication Research, 11*(1), 33–60.

Northouse, P. G., & Northouse, L. L. (1987). Communication about cancer: Issues confronting patients, health professional and family members. *Journal of Psychosocial Oncology, 5*(3), 17–46.

O'Hair, D. (1989). Dimensions of relational communication and control during physician–patient interactions. *Health Communication, 1*, 97–115.

Rogers, L. E., & Farace, R. V. (1975). Analysis of relational communication in dyads: New measurement procedures. *Human Communication Research, 3*, 222–239.

Roter, D. L., & Hall, J. A. (1989). Studies of doctor–patient interaction. *Annual Review of Public Health, 10*, 163–180.

Roter, D. L., & Hall, J. A. (1992). *Doctors talking with patients/patients talking with doctors: Improving communication in medical visits.* Westport, CT: Auburn.

Roter, D. L., Hall, J. A., & Katz, N. R. (1988). Patient–physician communication: A descriptive summary of the literature. *Patient Education and Counseling, 12*, 99–119.

Ruesch, J., & Bateson, G. (1951). *Communication: The social matrix of psychiatry.* New York: Norton.

Sluzki, G. E., & Beavin, J. (1965). Simetriay complementaridid: Una definicion operacional y una tipologia de parejas [Symmetry and complementarity: An operational definition and a typology of dyads]. *Acta Psiquiatrica y Psicologica de America Latina, 11*, 321–330.

Spitzberg, B. H., & Hecht, M. L. (1984). A component model of relational competence. *Human Communication Research, 10*, 575–600.

Stewart, M. A., & Weston, W. W. (1995). Introduction. In M. Stewart, J. B. Brown, W. W. Weston, I. R. McWhinney, & C. L. Freeman (Eds.), *Patient-centered medicine: Transforming the clinical method* (pp. xv–xxiv). Thousand Oaks, CA: Sage.

Stiles, W. B. (1989). Evaluating medical interview process components: Null corrections with outcomes may be misleading. *Medical Care, 27*, 212–220.

Street, R. L., Jr. (1992). Analyzing communication in medical consultations: Do behavioral measures correspond to patients' perceptions? *Medical Care, 30*, 976–988.

Tate, P. (1983). Doctor's style. In D. Pendleton & J. Hasler (Eds.), *Doctor–patient communication* (pp. 75–85). London: Academic.

von Friederichs-Fitzwater, M. M., Callahan, E. J., Flynn, N., & Williams, J. (1991). Relational control in physician–patient encounters. *Health Communication, 3*, 17–36.

Waitzkin, H. (1991). *The politics of medical encounters.* New Haven, CT: Yale University Press.

Watzlawick, P., Beavin, J., & Jackson, D. D. (1967). *Pragmatics of human communication.* New York: Norton.

West, C. (1983). "Ask me no questions ... :" An analysis of queries and replies in physician–patient dialogues. In S. Fisher & A. D. Todd (Eds.), *The social organization of doctor–patient communication* (pp. 55–74). Washington, DC: Center for Applied Linguistics.

Weston, W. W., & Brown, J. B. (1995). Dealing with common difficulties in learning and teaching the patient-centered method. In M. Stewart, J. B. Brown, W. W. Weston, I. R. McWhinney, & C. L. Freeman (Eds.), *Patient-centered medicine: Transforming the clinical method* (pp. 132–143). Thousand Oaks, CA: Sage.

Wigginton, D. (1995). *Relational control patterns in physician–patient clinical encounters.* Unpublished doctoral dissertation, University of Utah, Salt Lake City.

Wilmot, W. W. (1980). *Dyadic communication.* Menlo Park, CA: Addison-Wesley.

## APPENDIX A
### Message Coding

| 1st Digit (Speaker) | 2nd Digit (Message Format) | 3rd Digit (Response Mode) |
|---|---|---|
| 1 = physician | 1 = assertion | 1 = support |
| 2 = patient | 2 = question | 2 = support |
| | 3 = talk over | 3 = extension |
| | 4 = noncomplete | 4 = answer |
| | 5 = other | 5 = instruction |
| | 6 = silence | 6 = order |
| | | 7 = disconfirmation |
| | | 8 = topic change |
| | | 9 = termination |
| | | 0 = other |

## APPENDIX B
### Patient Demographics

| File No. | Patient Gender | Age | Ethnicity | Marital Status | Income | Education |
|---|---|---|---|---|---|---|
| 904 | Female | 22 | White | Divorced | > $10,000 | 12th grade |
| 906 | Female | 23 | White | Married | $10,000–$20,000 | 16th grade |
| 911 | Female | 19 | White | Separated | $10,000–$20,000 | 11th grade |
| 917 | Male | 38 | Black | Divorced | $20,000–$30,000 | 13th grade |
| 931 | Female | 27 | Hispanic | Separated | $10,000–$20,000 | 12th grade |
| 941 | Female | 36 | Hispanic | Single | $10,000–$20,000 | 11th grade |
| 947 | Female | 23 | White | Married | > $10,000 | 12th grade |
| 948 | Male | 69 | Black | Married | $10,000–$20,000 | 5th grade |
| 954 | Male | 43 | White | Single | > $10,000 | 16th grade |
| 955 | Male | 53 | Black | Separated | > $10,000 | 8th grade |

## RESPONSES

# Analyzing the Physician–Patient Interaction: An Overview of Six Methods and Future Research Directions

Rajiv N. Rimal

*Department of Communication Studies*
*The University of Texas*

The six research teams highlighted in this special issue of *Health Communication* were concerned with developing a methodologically sound and theoretically heuristic coding scheme to document the provider–patient interaction, and all articles coded the same set of provider–patient interactions. In this article, I first summarize the similarities and differences among the six articles and then raise two fundamental questions that are designed to stimulate further research in the field.

## COMPARISON OF THE SIX STUDIES

A striking aspect of this overall project is the wide diversity in the methods developed and tested by the research teams. Four of the six studies[1] (Studies 1, 3, 4, and 6), for example, coded all utterances in the medical interviews, one (Study 5) coded only utterances that indicated physician or patient participation, and one (Study 2) made global assessments of physician talk from the perspective of patients. Researchers varied widely even in quantifying the total number of utterances per interview: 392 (Study 1), 694 (Study 3), 730 (Study 4), and 591 (Study 6). That research-

Requests for reprints should be sent to Rajiv N. Rimal, Department of Communication Studies, The University of Texas, Austin, TX 78712. E-mail: rimal@mail.utexas.edu

[1]For the sake of brevity, the six studies in this special issue are referred to (in alphabetical order) as Study 1 (McNeilis), Study 2 (Meredith, Stewart, & Brown), Study 3 (Roter & Larson), Study 4 (Shaikh, Knobloch, & Stiles), Study 5 (Street & Millay), and Study 6 (von Friederichs-Fitzwater & Gilgun).

ers used different methods may be understandable, given that the six teams were chosen on the basis of their own expertise. We can certainly construe it as indicative of the rich diversity in our field—an example of how the same phenomenon can be studied in multiple ways. If, however, different methods lead to different conclusions, we might argue that the field has yet been unable to agree on how to develop reliable and valid coding schemes that transcend individual researchers' interests and speak to larger issues. Study 5 found, for example, that only a small portion (1.5%) of physician talk was patient centered, but Study 2 concluded the opposite. Two studies (Studies 3 and 6) reported a preponderance of doctor-centered or disease-centered pattern of interactions, and two studies (Studies 1 and 4) warned against drawing such conclusions on a global basis; rather, they showed that patterns vary widely according to the segment (Study 4) as well as the goal (Study 1) of the medical interview.

Apart from the diversity of methods used by the research teams, differential findings can also be attributed to the wide range of contextual factors considered important in each study. Study 2, for example, made global assessments without taking contextual factors into account, which resulted in substantially different findings. Contextual factors important in Study 1 were utterances that preceded and followed the utterance under investigation, whereas the most important contextual factor in Study 4 was the segment of the medical interview. Study 3 distinguished residents from attending physicians and Study 6 was concerned with the impact of differences in power in determining the nature of the communication in the medical encounter. Finally, Study 5 was the only one that made assessments both qualitatively and quantitatively.

The principal finding to emerge from the six studies was the idea of control. In concordance with the existing literature, Studies 1, 4, and 6 found that physicians exerted greater control than patients, but Studies 5 and 6 reported that patients could benefit from assertiveness—patient queries were seldom ignored by physicians, who participated in greater partnership-building communication when patients themselves were engaged. In the next section, by raising two questions, I explore how the six studies conceptualized communication and how research can benefit from other interpretations of the communication between physicians and patients.

## QUESTION 1:
## WHAT IS THE UNDERLYING DEFINITION
## OF COMMUNICATION?

An assumption across the six featured studies in particular and in the larger field of physician–patient communication in general is that communication is at the heart of the matter—that positive outcomes result from better and more effective communication between physicians and patients. Indeed, a long tradition of research in this area points to the benefits of improved communication on the part of both physicians (Ramirez, Graham, Richards, Cull, & Gregory, 1996) and patients (Gotcher, 1995; see Stewart, 1995, for a review). Given this central assumption guiding the work on physician–patient communication, the first question I raise in this article is this: To the extent that the six articles featured in this special issue are representative of work in the larger field, how do researchers conceptualize communication?

To answer this question, I turn to Carey's (1989) distinction between the transmission and ritualistic views of communication. According to Carey, the *transmission view* defines communication as "a process whereby messages are transmitted and distributed in space for the control of distance and people" (p. 15). In this view, communication is used as an instrument for achieving a desired end. Using this conceptualization, we can interpret patients' talk as being guided by their desires to be properly diagnosed and treated for diseases, and physicians' talk as being guided by their desire to properly diagnose and treat diseases. *Ritualistic communication,* on the other hand, is concerned not with "the act of imparting information," but "the representation of shared beliefs," and it "draws persons together in fellowship and commonality" (Carey, 1989, p. 18). This view is analogous to "attending a mass, a situation in which nothing new is learned but in which a particular view of the world is portrayed and confirmed" (Carey, 1989, p. 20). Hence, the transmission view conceptualizes communication in terms of extrinsic, and the ritualistic view in terms of intrinsic, goals.

This distinction is obviously meant for heuristic purposes only, and it is not to be construed as a mutually exclusive categorization. Research on provider–patient interaction, however, is predominantly concerned with the transmission view of communication. It assumes that the verbal exchange between the physician and the patient is meant to fulfill goals that are external to the interaction. Given that the purpose of most visitations is to fulfill some health-related need of the patient, this orientation toward the transmission view of communication is understandable. However, if human communication consists of both components, we have to ask what we are neglecting in our research by ignoring the ritualistic aspect.

Consider Study 4, which categorizes the medical visitation into three segments—medical history, physical examination, and conclusion. Adopting the transmission view, the authors show that goals of the physician–patient communication vary according to the segment of the visitation. During the medical history segment, for example, physicians are attentive, whereas patients are informative, and this segment mainly comprises patients' attempts, via communication, to make the physician understand the nature of their medical problem. However, one could also interpret many of the actions performed by physicians and patients according to the ritualistic view—that in the initial medical history segment, patients and physicians alike follow certain rules and formalities they have internalized through their past experiences in similar situations. To the extent that these rituals are performed, both parties are likely to find comfort in the interaction. Indeed, research from psychotherapy indicates that rituals can act to improve the collaboration between the client and therapist (Al-Krenawi, 1999).[2] Following prescribed rituals can alleviate anxieties on the part of patients, who may find comfort in familiar routines. Physicians' failure, for whatever reason, to follow established rituals is likely to induce anxieties on the part of patients. Rituals may be broken, for example, if physicians do not sequentially follow the three (medical history, physical examination, and conclusion) segments as outlined in Study 4 or if they inappropriately emphasize characteristics of one segment while functioning in another.

## Research Implications of Adopting the Ritualistic View

A focus on the ritualistic view has potentially important implications for how we interpret exchanges that take place between physicians and patients, and more research in this area is certainly needed. We know little, for example, about the kinds of rituals inherent in a physician–patient exchange: whether they are related to patient perceptions and outcomes, whether they differ according to physicians' and patients' characteristics, and whether they change over time. Application of the ritualistic aspect of communication can help us understand the representations individuals have of health and illness (Farr & Markova, 1995), and we can view the physician–patient interaction as an ongoing narrative, one in which health issues are discussed in the larger context of individuals' lives (Kleinman, 1988; Sharf, 1990). We can then develop a typology of rituals inherent in the physician–patient interaction, as have researchers who study other relationships, including marriage (Baxter & Dindia, 1990; Berg-Cross, Daniels, & Carr, 1992), family (Bossard & Bole, 1950), and adult friendships (Bruess & Pearson, 1997).

Another fruitful area of research lies in conceptualizing the physician–patient interaction in terms of the scripts that both parties follow during their exchange. Interactions in which we participate on a regular basis follow scripts we have internalized through similar past (real or vicarious) experiences. Some researchers have already begun conceptualizing individuals' health behaviors in terms of the scripts they employ to negotiate meaning with others. De Zwart, van Kerkhof, and Sandfort (1998), for example, studied the sexual behavior among gay men, and they identified four distinct scenarios that provided structure and meaning to the use of condoms during anal sex: the physical (in which condoms were seen as ob-

---

[2]Goffman (1967) defined *rituals* as "acts through whose symbolic component the actor shows how worthy he is of respect or how worthy he feels others are of it" (p. 19). A definition of rituals closer to the field of communication is provided by Bruess and Pearson (1997): "Stylized, repetitive, communicative enactments that pay homage to a valued object, person, or phenomenon" (p. 25).

stacles to bodily pleasure), the intimate (hindrance to emotional closeness), the reciprocal (disruption for each act of sexual pleasure), and power (facilitation for the integration of condom use). A similar technique could be used to study the physician–patient interaction.

To study the physician–patient interaction according to a ritualistic view of communication we have to shift our unit of analysis from the individual (be it the patient or the physician) to the dyad. This is illustrated in Study 6, which conceptualized the physician–patient interaction according to a relational control methodology in which the central issue revolves around power—which of the two interactants attempts to exert control. This emphasis on the dyad is not to suggest that individual characteristics are unimportant. Indeed, it is quite likely that the repertoire of scripts and strategies at individuals' disposal is a function of their personalities and past experiences. Those with a long history of medical visitations are likely to have a variety of negotiation strategies at their disposal and, conversely, those with little prior experience, because of their unfamiliarity with the medical visitation rituals, are likely to be constrained in their interactions (Greene, 1990). An interesting hypothesis that emerges from this argument is that the variety of prior experiences of patients and physicians will collectively determine the quality of their mutual interaction. After all, those who have a rich repertoire of prior experiences are able to draw from both a wider selection of internalized negotiation strategies as well as the outcomes of those strategies (Greene, 1984; Street, 1997). This further implies that research on physician–patient interactions has to incorporate both parties' prior experiences if we are to gain a richer understanding of the communicative processes.

Power and control comprise only one set of concepts that arise from a focus on the dyad as the unit of analysis. Scholars (e.g., Baxter, 1988; Montgomery, 1992; Rawlins, 1992) have developed other concepts, including the idea of dialectics, tensions, or contradictions that individuals negotiate in interpersonal relationships. Baxter (1988) noted, for example, that contradictions are formed "whenever two tendencies or forces are interdependent yet mutually negate one another" (p. 258), and she classified tensions according to whether they are internal (negotiated within the relationship) or external (imposed from the outside). These tensions provide an opportunity for individuals to negotiate their identity within the broader context of the relationship, and Baxter (1990) provided six strategies (selection, cyclic alternation, segmentation, moderation, disqualification, and reframing) that individuals use to do so.

Our study of physician–patient interactions could benefit immensely if we draw from extant work on interpersonal relationships. In a broad theoretical context, we could ask questions about the extent to which dialectics in the physician–patient interaction mirror those documented in other (e.g., intimate) interpersonal relationships. For example, what are some of the dialectics or tensions faced by both physicians and patients and what strategies do they use to negotiate a mutually acceptable resolution? Expanding on the tension between self-disclosure and privacy, Baxter (1988) noted that individuals negotiate their internal desires for privacy with the interpersonal demands for openness. This seems to be a highly relevant concept with which to analyze the physician–patient communication.

Many of the suggestions for future research that I have pointed out thus far lend themselves to qualitative analyses. This is not to negate the value of quantitative methods. On the contrary, readers can note for themselves the excellent contribution that researchers included in this special issue have made to the literature on physician–patient communication by using quantitative techniques. Rather, a healthy fusion of both methods, as shown, for example, in Study 5, would add both breadth and depth to our intellectual pursuits.

## QUESTION 2:
## WHOSE PERSPECTIVE ARE WE STUDYING
## AND WHOSE PERSPECTIVE MATTERS?

The same communication situation can be viewed from the perspective of multiple stakeholders, including that of the health care administration, the physician, and the patient. Each of these perspectives can lead to a substantially different evaluation of the same interaction because, for example, the issues relevant to each of these stakeholders are likely to be different. Into this myriad of (often) competing interests enter the researchers with their own perspectives.

Relative to the number of studies that adopt either the physicians' or the patients' perspectives, there is sparse literature on how the physician–patient communication process is influenced by the perspective of the institutional providers. Perhaps the absence of an institutional-centered focus in the literature reflects an underlying desire on the part of researchers to adopt a patient–advocate role. However, ignoring the most powerful stakeholder's perspective can lead to a number of consequences. First, our efforts to secure a meaningful dialogue, one based on a comprehensive analysis of the communication process among all stakeholders, is likely to be limited. Second, as long as our research agenda continues to neglect institutional issues, we are likely to constrain our inquiries to ones that take for granted the institutionally imposed boundary conditions. Hence, changes we advocate are likely to be restricted to those that can be undertaken at the individual (e.g., the physician or patient), rather than at the institutional, level. Third, it is difficult to imagine how the extant ideology of health care provision can be changed in the absence of a focus on the larger issues that determine the behavior of both the physicians and patients as a function of institutional characteristics.

What are some of the communication-related research questions we might raise if we are to incorporate larger institutional issues into our research agenda? One set of questions could concentrate on the institutional constraints imposed on both the patient and the physician. We might ask questions, for example, about the relationship between the length of time spent and the bureaucracy encountered by patients before they are able to see the physician, on the one hand, and the nature of the physician–patient communication experience, on the other. To the extent that institutional bureaucracies impinge on patients' decision-making processes, it is likely that patients' perceptions about their abilities to become equal partners in the medical encounter and their willingness to communicate with their physicians will both suffer. Institutional constraints are also likely to affect physicians' willingness to communicate effectively with their patients. To what extent, for example, are physicians guided by institutional demands on their time? It is likely that institutional guidelines for increasing the efficiency of each visit (defined in terms of the number of patients seen per unit time) will impinge on physicians' communication activities with their patients (Ben-Sira, 1990). By focusing exclusively on either the physicians' or the patients' perspective, researchers are likely to neglect these external factors that impinge on the physician–patient communication.

By adopting either the physician's or the patient's perspective, the research articles included in this issue have already addressed the various topics likely to be of concern to both parties. Indeed, the reciprocal relationship between physicians and patients has been the focus of much of the literature in the field. Whereas earlier work adopted the physician's perspective, the more recent trend has been to study the patient's role (Byrne & Long, 1984; Stewart, 1995). Researchers who study the patient's perspective have pointed out the limitations associated with adopting only the physician's perspective in our research (Geist & Dreyer, 1993; Levenstein, McCracken, McWhinney, Stewart, & Brown, 1986). This has led many researchers to advocate a patient-empowerment model, one in which the patients, relative to physicians, are seen as equal partners in a mutual interaction (Levenstein et al., 1986; for a review, see Street, 2001).

The underlying premise among researchers advocating a patient-empowerment model is that patients are better served to the extent they become equal participants in their medical decision-making process. Inherent in this argument is the assumption that, by default, patients either do not actively participate in decision making or that they are unable to do so because of constraints imposed on them by medical institutions, physicians, or their own cognitive or behavioral limitations. Missing from this patient empowerment model are considerations about patients' desire to participate actively in the decision-making process. Whereas we have been inquiring about how we can improve patient participation, we also need to ask whether patients want to become equal participants (vis à vis their physicians) in decision making. We have been characterizing physician-centered communication models as "paternalistic" because they impose values of the powerful (e.g., physicians) on the powerless (patients). Can we not characterize the imposition of researchers' values on patients similarly? After all, patient empowerment models are built on the premise that patients should want to participate in their medical decisions.

These models may well capture the desires of a majority of patients. If so, informing patients about their rights and responsibilities and improving their decision-making competencies seem to be viable strategies (Rimal, Ratzan, Arnston, & Freimuth, 1997). If, however, some patients would prefer to defer medical decisions to their providers (Ende, Kazis, Ash, & Moskowitz, 1989; Strull, Lo, & Charles, 1984), whom they consider to be more knowledgeable or competent than themselves, should we, as researchers or patient advocates, continue to insist on "educating" patients to the contrary? Consider the research reported by Strull et al., who examined hypertensive patients' perceptions about their involvement in decision making. Whereas a majority (63%) of the patients reported that decisions were usually made by the clinician, less than a quarter of the sample reported that they wanted to become equal participants in the decision-making process. Given these findings, how do our patient empowerment models interpret situations where patients decide not to decide?

This is an important issue to consider for a number of reasons. First, from an ethical perspective, we as researchers and practitioners have to respect the desires and wishes of those on whose behalf we wish to intervene. To the extent that patients wish to defer decisions to their providers, interventions to the contrary are not only unethical, in the long run they are bound to be counterproductive. Second, to the extent we assume all patients wish to participate in decision making, we are likely to adopt a "blame the victim" attitude when outcomes do not conform to our expectations. Third, because patients may not possess the technical expertise to fully understand the consequences of their choices, interventions that are only concerned with improving patients' communicative competencies (without also improving medical knowledge, for example) are likely to foster an illusion of control. Such interventions are likely to fail if, to begin with, patients have little motivation to actively participate in the decision-making process.

## A Typology of Participation

To the extent that patients' desires to abdicate control are due to their poor communicative competencies, interventions that seek to improve those competencies could assist patients in making informed decisions about participating in their medical care. However, we cannot take it as a given that improving communicative competencies will result in greater participation. Based on patients' abilities and desires to participate,[3] we can define four distinct groups: (a) *constrained,* or

---

[3] By *ability,* I mean patients' real or perceived communication competencies, which includes knowledge about what needs to be communicated as well as the skills to translate knowledge into action. As pointed out in Study 1, competencies can also be conceptualized according to the two general goals—informational and relational—inherent in interpersonal exchanges. These goals also correspond to the transmission view and the ritualistic view of communication, respectively.

those who wish but are unable to participate in decision making; (b) *active,* or those who wish and are able to participate; (c) *passive,* or those who neither wish nor are able to participate; and (d) *restrained,* or those who do not wish but are able to participate. Once we categorize patients into one of these four groups, we can begin to recognize that different research questions as well as different interventions will be relevant for each of the four groups. For example, research questions directed at the constrained group may be concerned with barriers that prevent individuals from participating. Research shows, for example, that a variety of factors, including perceived norms about the appropriateness of taking too much of the provider's time (Roter & Hall, 1993; Street, 2001) and internal locus of control (Howell-Koren & Tinsley, 1990), prevent patients from participating in their medical encounters. It would thus appear that cognitive restructuring strategies, ones designed to change individuals' normative perceptions, would work best for this group. Research questions most relevant for the active group might include, Do individuals in this group actually participate and how can interventions facilitate participation? Because individuals in the passive group neither wish nor are able to participate in medical decision making, the most relevant research question in studying this group may be to ask if there is a causal relation between ability and desire. In other words, if the passive group's desire to refrain from participation is because of inabilities, then interventions designed to increase this group's communicative competencies would be most beneficial. However, if there is no relation between desire and ability, then researchers should accept and respect individuals' desires to abdicate control. Finally, individuals in the restrained group, despite their communicative competencies, do not wish to participate. For this group of patients, we might ask questions about their other concerns in the medical encounter. For example, patients may want to spend the least amount of time in a physician's office. If so, we might inquire about how their time could be utilized most efficiently.

These research questions are meant to be heuristic, not exhaustive. To begin work according to the typology just suggested, perhaps the first step is to tabulate descriptive statistics in terms of the distribution of individuals in the four groups. We may also want to determine if there are personality, cultural, and institutional factors that predispose individuals into one of the four aforementioned groups. I do not, however, wish to suggest that the four groups represent individual differences. It is conceivable, indeed quite likely, that membership into one of the four groups is situational. For example, communicatively competent individuals may desire not to spend much time with their medical providers when they want to receive a flu shot, but they may want extensive input from their physicians to make an intelligent decision about which cancer therapy is best for them. The broader point here is that we cannot, indeed should not, treat all individuals as if they are being constrained in actualizing their desires to fully participate in the medical encounter.

## CONCLUDING REMARKS

The six articles included in this special issue provide us with multiple perspectives on the physician–patient communication process. It is clear from these articles that the theoretical prism through which we view the medical encounter largely determines what we see. That different theoretical orientations lead to different results is not inherently problematic. It can be misleading, however, if we are not explicit about our assumptions and definitions. In this article, I focused on the two definitions of communication to illustrate how some of the underlying assumptions have guided our work in the field. I also attempted to highlight some areas of research that have not received adequate attention. Further, because communicative processes involve multiple perspectives that are mutually negotiated, I have also pointed out the importance of being explicit about whose perspective underlies our inquiries. Finally, it is important that we as researchers not allow our values to supersede those of patients'. Although adopting these recommendations will not necessarily lead to a convergence in future research findings, I do hope that the questions raised in this article will stimulate further thinking on how best to proceed.

## ACKNOWLEDGMENT

This article was written during the author's tenure at the Department of Speech Communication, Texas A&M University.

## REFERENCES

Al-Krenawi, A. (1999). An overview of rituals in Western therapies and intervention: Argument for their use in cross-cultural therapy. *International Journal for the Advancement of Counseling, 21,* 3–17.

Baxter, L. (1988). A dialectical perspective on communication strategies in relationship development. In S. Duck (Ed.), *A handbook of personal relationships* (pp. 257–273). New York: Wiley.

Baxter, L. (1990). Dialectical contradictions in relationship development. *Journal of Social and Personal Relationships, 7,* 69–88.

Baxter, L. A., & Dindia, K. (1990). Marital partners' perceptions of marital maintenance strategies. *Journal of Social and Personal Relationships, 7,* 187–208.

Ben-Sira, Z. (1990). Primary care practitioners' likelihood to engage in biopsychosocial approach: An additional perspective on the doctor–patient relationship. *Social Science and Medicine, 31,* 565–576.

Berg-Cross, L., Daniels, C., & Carr, P. (1992). Marital rituals among divorced and married couples. *Journal of Divorce and Remarriage, 18,* 1–30.

Bossard, J. H. S., & Bole, E. S. (1950). *Ritual in family living: A contemporary study.* Philadelphia: University of Pennsylvania Press.

Bruess, C. J. C., & Pearson, J. C. (1997). Interpersonal rituals in marriage and adult friendship. *Communication Monographs, 64,* 25–46.

Byrne, P. S., & Long, B. E. L. (1984). *Doctors talking to patients.* London: Royal College of General Practitioners.

Carey, J. W. (1989). *Communication as culture: Essays on media and society*. Boston: Unwin Hyman.

de Zwart, O., van Kerkhof, M. P. N., & Sandfort, T. G. M. (1998). Anal sex and gay men: The challenge of HIV and beyond. *Journal of Psychology and Human Sexuality, 10*, 89–102.

Ende, J., Kazis, L., Ash, A., & Moskowitz, M. A. (1989). Measuring patients' desire for autonomy: Decision-making and information-seeking preferences among medical patients. *Journal of General Internal Medicine, 4*, 23–30.

Farr, R. M., & Markova, I. (1995). Professional and lay representations of health, illness and handicap: A theoretical overview. In I. Markova & R. M. Farr (Eds.), *Representations of health, illness and handicap* (pp. 93–110). London: Harwood.

Geist, P., & Dreyer, J. (1993). The demise of dialogue: A critique of medical encounter dialogue. *Western Journal of Communication, 57*, 233–246.

Goffman, E. (1967). *Interaction ritual: Essays in face-to-face behavior*. Chicago: Aldine.

Gotcher, J. M. (1995). Well-adjusted and maladjusted cancer patients: An examination of communication variables. *Health Communication, 7*, 21–33.

Greene, J. O. (1984). A cognitive approach to human communication: An action assembly theory. *Communication Monographs, 51*, 289–306.

Greene, J. O. (1990). Tactical social action: Towards some strategies for theory. In M. J. Cody & M. L. McLaughlin (Eds.), *The psychology of tactical communication* (pp. 31–47). Clevendon, PA: Multilingual Matters.

Howell-Koren, P. R., & Tinsley, B. J. (1990). The relationships among maternal health locus of control beliefs and expectations, pediatrician–mother communication, and maternal satisfaction with well-infant care. *Health Communication, 2*, 233–253.

Kleinman, A. (1988). *The illness narratives: Suffering, healing, and the human condition*. New York: Basic Books.

Levenstein, J. H., McCracken, E. C., McWhinney, I. R., Stewart, M. A., & Brown, J. B. (1986). The patient-centered clinical method: 1. A model for the doctor–patient interaction in family medicine. *Family Practice, 3*, 24–30.

Montgomery, B. (1992). Communication as the interface between couples and culture. In S. Deetz (Ed.), *Communication yearbook* (pp. 475–507). Newbury Park, CA: Sage.

Ramirez, A. J., Graham, J., Richards, M. A., Cull, A., & Gregory, W. M. (1996). Mental health of hospital consultants: The effects of stress and satisfaction at work. *Lancet, 347*, 724–729.

Rawlins, W. (1992). *Friendship matters: Communication, dialectics, and the life course*. New York: Aldine de Gruyter.

Rimal, R. N., Ratzan, S. C., Arnston, P., & Freimuth, V. S. (1997). Reconceptualizing the "patient": Health care promotion as increasing citizens' decision-making competencies. *Health Communication, 9*, 61–74.

Roter, D. L., & Hall, J. A. (1993). *Doctors talking with patients/patients talking with doctors*. Westport, CT: Auburn.

Sharf, B. F. (1990). Physician–patient communication as interpersonal rhetoric: A narrative approach. *Health Communication, 2*, 217–232.

Stewart, M. A. (1995). Effective physician–patient communication and health outcomes: A review. *Canadian Medical Association Journal, 152*, 1423–1433.

Street, R. L., Jr. (1997). Methodological considerations when assessing communication skills. *Medical Encounter, 13*, 3–7.

Street, R. L., Jr. (2001). Active patients as powerful communicators: The linguistic foundation of participation in health care. In W. P. Robinson & H. Giles (Eds.), *The new handbook of language and social psychology* (pp. 541–560). Chichester, England: Wiley.

Strull, W. M., Lo, B., & Charles, G. (1984). Do patients want to participate in medical decision-making? *Journal of the American Medical Association, 252*, 2990–2994.

# Cracking the Code: Theory and Method in Clinical Communication Analysis

Richard M. Frankel

*The Fetzer Institute*
*Kalamazoo, Michigan*

In 1971, and based on work originally begun at Stanford University in 1955, an interdisciplinary group of social scientists (McQuown, Bateson, Birdwhistell, Brosen, & Hockett, 1971) completed a massive study of a single interview titled "The Natural History of an Interview." Each member of the team had been given a copy of the 16-mm film on which the interview had been captured and each analyzed it according to their own particular point of view. The completed manuscript from the project ran more than 700 pages. Although it is available on University of Chicago microfilm, the study was never published, in part, because like blind men describing an elephant, there was little overall cohesiveness to the analysis and little agreement on what it all meant.

Some 3 decades later we find this special issue of *Health Communication* based on an analysis of 10 routine primary care visits in a teaching clinic. Using a procedure similar to McQuown et al.'s (1971), each of the investigators chosen to contribute an article to the issue received a videotape copy of the 10 encounters and were invited to analyze them according to their particular interests and frameworks. The result is a fascinating look at the various ways scholarship has developed in studying doctor–patient communication, the different assumptions each system of analysis employs, and the different conclusions that each yields because everyone analyzed the same data. Happily, the results of this undertaking are being published (in fewer than 700 pages!) and provide a useful point of departure for understanding how a field of study develops and matures over time.

Before commenting on the particulars of the studies in this issue, I provide a historical framework for understanding these and other studies of physician–patient communication. In so doing, I hope to draw attention to a creative tension that

Requests for reprints should be sent to Richard M. Frankel, Vice President for Program Evaluation, The Fetzer Institute, 9292 KL Avenue, Kalamazoo, MI 49009. E-mail: rfrankel@fetzer.org

exists among methodologists about how best to study clinical interaction. My conclusion is that the "best" way to study any problem depends on the question that is being asked and the tools and resources that are available to study it.

## TWO APPROACHES TO STUDYING DOCTOR–PATIENT COMMUNICATION AND TWO WORLDVIEWS

In the late 1930s, psychiatrists W. F. Murphy and Felix Deutch began making wire recordings of visits between psychiatric residents and their patients. The purpose of making these recordings was to create "a sound mirror" as it were, to provide feedback and instruction to trainees. Stoeckle and Billings (1987) identified this early educational practice as the beginning of the modern era in studying the medical encounter. Since that time, the idea of capturing interviewing performance on a stable and reproducible medium (audio, video, film), and representing and analyzing it, has grown in popularity and has produced impressive results (Stewart, 1995; Stewart et al., 1999).

Two schools of thought exist on how interactional material should be handled methodologically. The first school is concerned with preserving as much as possible of the details of an interaction and the moment by moment changes that take place as it progresses. Investigators in this tradition use film frames, live drawings, and elaborate transcription systems to capture key performance elements or moments often from a single interaction. Intensive attention is paid to the most minute details of the interaction and it may be replayed and reviewed hundreds, even thousands of times to achieve a deep understanding of the form of the interaction and how individuals participate in it. (For a comprehensive review of the foundations of this type of interaction analysis, see Jordan & Henderson, 1995.)

In this tradition it is not uncommon for investigators to spend years and create incredibly detailed analyses of surprisingly short interactional episodes. Pittinger, Hockett, and Danehy (1960), for example, published an entire monograph based on the first 5 min of a recorded interaction. Similarly, Sheflen (1971) published a 375-page monograph that took him 10 years to complete analyzing the interaction in a 30-min psychiatric encounter. Others such as Condon and Ogston (1967, 1971) have done frame-by-frame analysis of synchronized motion between newborns and their mothers and later speakers and hearers using time lapses as short as 0.001 sec. An entire analysis might take 10 sec in clock time and contain 10,000 frames or data points, each of which is individually analyzed. Much like the early microscopists whose evidence consisted of directly observing and drawing images of specimens observed under magnification and whose results led to an understanding of life at the cellular level, the tradition of recording and representing the details of social life directly has led to some fundamental reconceptualizations of what it means to be human and to be in helping as well as other types of relationships.

## In Another Galaxy Far Away ...

About the same time that interaction in clinical encounters was being analyzed in ever increasing detail, another group of researchers was struggling with a different, but equally important set of problems—to evaluate the real time interactional dynamics of small groups such as classrooms, work groups, and encounters between professionals and clients. There is a rich intellectual history surrounding the development of small group interaction analysis and the modifications that have been made by various scholars who have adopted it for doctor–patient communication studies. For our purposes in this short article it is important to remember that (a) researchers during this time period were looking for cost effective ways of analyzing multiple interactions in real time, and (b) to be useful as an evaluation tool, the analytic scheme had to be able to produce valid, reliable, and generalizable results.

With these challenges in mind, Bales (1950), a statistician in the Department of Social Relations at Harvard, developed a coding scheme which married his own work on small group dynamics with that of Parsons, the dominant sociological theorist of the time, and also a colleague in the Department of Social Relations.

The heart of Bales's (1950) coding system is what Parsons and Shills (1952) termed a *pattern variable,* which was defined as a

dichotomy one side of which must be chosen by an actor before the meaning of a situation is determinant for him, and thus before he can act with respect to that situation. We maintain that there are only five *basic* pattern variables ... they constitute a [social] system.

In essence, Parsons and Bales claimed that a very limited number of pattern variables could be used to create an exhaustive, mutually exclusive system for coding the most salient dimensions of social interaction in small groups. Bales's (1950) system has had an impressive life span and continues to be used by researchers in a variety of settings from classrooms to the e-mail correspondence on the Internet.

In the medical context a variety of modifications have been made to Bales's (1950) original system. In the late 1960s, Barbara Korsch, a pediatrician at the University of Southern California conducted a number of pioneering studies of pediatrician–patient–parent interactions using a modified version of Bales's system that allowed for additional communication dimensions such as information giving and advice to be coded (Korsch, Gozzi, & Frances, 1968; Korsch & Negrete, 1972). Shortly after Korsch's work appeared, Barbara Starfield (Starfield et al., 1979; Starfield et al., 1981), also a pediatrician at John's Hopkins University, further modified the scheme to include such things as agreement on the nature of the problem and the proposed solution. In the late 1970s, Debra Roter, who had been a student of Starfield's at Hopkins, modified the system further and devised the Roter Interactional Analysis Scale (RIAS; Roter, 1977). Like Bales's scheme, the RIAS is based on pattern variable and polar typologies. Unlike his system, the RIAS is sensitive to some of the unique characteristics of physician–patient interaction such as dominance (as measured by who asks and who answers questions in the encounter). On the basis of her early analyses, Roter designed an intervention to test the efficacy of teaching patients to become more assertive in the encounter by asking more questions. It was her finding that this intervention improved health care outcomes such as satisfaction and adherence that won her doctoral dissertation a national award in 1977. The RIAS has been in continuous use since.

In trying to sharpen the focus around the two research traditions, it is useful to think of researchers in the first tradition attempting to achieve a naturalistic or photographic representation of phenomena as the basis for analysis. By contrast, researchers in the second tradition strive to represent interactional events at a higher level of abstraction using terms that are valid, reliable, and comparable. In the same way that a map and a photograph represent the same terrain in different ways and for different purposes so too do the tools for studying clinical interaction. As such, they stand not so much in opposition to one another as they address different needs and concerns. For a more in depth treatment of this idea, see Roter and Frankel (1992).

Five of the six articles that make up this special issue fall squarely into the tradition of coding interaction. (The contribution by Street & Millay nicely integrates methods from both traditions.) The predominant focus, however, is on finding valid and reproducible ways of categorizing events and comparing within and between cases. The most significant variation in the different approaches has to do with the units of analysis adopted by each researcher and the extent to which the coding system is general purpose or "targeted."

For example, in their article, Shaikh, Knobloch, and Stiles define their *verbal response mode* (VRM) coding scheme as a "general purpose classification of speech acts" (this issue, p. 53). It measures three bipolar dimensions of social relationships: attentiveness versus informativeness, directness versus acquiescence, and presumptuousness versus unassumingness. Drawing on Parson's (1951) description of the physician's role as high status and controlling vis-à-vis the patient, Shaikh et al. ask the question of whether this role relation is fixed or whether it varies according to the different tasks that make up the encounter. The value of asking this question is that it potentially affects the norms that define what might be appropriate and effective for a given subcomponent of the encounter. Based on the eight complete visits from the data set, Shaikh et al. derived quantitative indexes of physician and patient roles and found significant differences in each of the three components studied (history, physical exam, conclusion). As the authors point out, the findings themselves are predictable in light of the tasks to be completed in each phase. What is important is that theorists and researchers who conceptualize the physician–patient relationship in global terms, without considering systematic changes in roles during the medical interview, may overlook a crucial aspect of the relationship. ... For example, aggregated profiles might make a physician appear to be exceptionally directive and presumptuous with patients whose condition required an unusually extended physical examination. (this issue, p. 59)

Like Shaikh et al.'s general purpose approach, the article contributed by Roter and Larson focuses on an application of the RIAS to the 10 taped encounters. The point of departure for this analysis was that, in addition to the resident and patient, 8 of the 10 encounters also involved a faculty preceptor who participated in them for relatively brief periods of time. Using the RIAS coding, Roter and Larson were interested in knowing how the faculty interactions with patients differed from those of the residents. They found a number of interesting patterns. For example, residents were relatively high in their biomedical focus, a finding consistent with other studies of young physicians. Surprisingly, attending physicians tended to be highly biomedical in terms of their contribution to the dialogue, were more engaged in probing residents' opinions and thought processes in the biomedical domain, and were less verbally engaged in more psychosocial visits. This is an important finding from an educational point of view because it suggests that attendings may verbally reinforce exploration on the biomedical side but disengage verbally when it comes to psychosocial issues. Whatever the reason it is worth further exploration in a larger sample, as the authors point out.

Two observations are worth noting about these studies. First, as general-purpose schemes, both the VRM and the RIAS are neutral with respect to what they may uncover and what it means. In terms of prospective research this is an advantage. The second observation speaks to the need to be explicit in terms of what is included or excluded for analysis. The substance of Roter and Larson's analysis is a comparison of communication styles in visits where an attending physician is present in a teaching capacity. The fact that 8 of the 10 visits included a third party attending is not even mentioned in Shaikh et al.'s description of the data set. Such an omission is understandable given the nature of the question the investigators were pursuing. However, it is possible that the residents' expectations of being precepted by their attending could have changed their behavior during the encounters. If so, this would represent an unacknowledged influence on the analytic results. Without access to the raw data it would be difficult to know that each analysis came from the same data set.

In contrast with Shaikh et al.'s and Roter and Larson's general-purpose schemes, the remaining four articles in this special issue use interaction coding to target communication behaviors that have been shown in clinical or nonclinical settings to be desirable in some way. Such criterion-based approaches are familiar to evaluation researchers whose goal is to judge performance against a "gold standard." Meredith,

Stewart, and Brown's article is a good case in point. Over the past 15 years the authors have developed and tested a model of clinical care called the *patient-centered clinical method*. There is convincing evidence from these studies that patient centeredness is associated with positive outcomes of care such as satisfaction, adherence, and resolution of symptoms (Stewart, 1995). As Meredith et al. point out, one of the main advantages of the scheme is that "it is theory based, that is, it was developed specifically to assess the behaviors of patients and doctors ascribed by the patient-centered clinical method (Stewart, 1995)" (this issue, p. 19).

It is interesting to compare how Meredith et al. handled the problem of inclusion or exclusion both of cases and of the presence of the preceptor in 8 of the 10 encounters. According to their description, Interview 4 has been omitted as per instructions of the editor. Interview 5 has also been omitted due to the fact that it is incomplete—the tape stops before the end of the interview. The patient-centered scoring method cannot be used on incomplete interviews. Across the six articles it is easy to see that there are different criteria employed for including or excluding cases, including directions from the editor. The lack of uniformity in how these issues are handled potentially creates ambiguity over whether the data, analysis, and conclusions are actually comparable.

On the other hand, to Meredith et al.'s credit, the complexity of precepting encounters, and the fact that their coding scheme had never been used to evaluate them before led this team to interpret the results with caution and suggest that changes will have to be made to the coding scheme to accommodate situations in which additional parties beyond the individual physician and patient are present and participating in the encounter.

The studies in the articles by von Friederichs-Fitzwater and Gilgun, and McNeilis illustrate attempts to translate communication concepts that have been found to be desirable or effective in contexts outside of clinical medicine and apply them to the recorded encounters. The two concepts are relational control, which has been widely used to study informal dyads such as couples, marital pairs, and family and work pairs, and communication competence, which is based on how well interactants manage content, alignment, and function within and across an encounter.

In their analysis of the taped encounters, von Friederichs-Fitzwater and Gilgun report on "10 physician–patient interactions [that] were videotaped and transcribed for coding and analysis. The interactions were first time visits by patients in a family practice clinic in an urban teaching medical center" (pp. 77–78). No additional information about inclusion or exclusion criteria or proportion of visits in which a teaching attending was present is reported. Using Roter and Larson's approach it would be very interesting to compare patterns of relational control in the conversations between the patient and each physician and the physicians themselves. Perhaps the same complexity experienced by Meredith et al. in their study and the fact that the coding scheme has primarily been used in dyads precluded this type of analysis. Whatever the case, the description of the data glosses the fact that additional parties were present in the majority of the encounters and that one encounter was not complete.

The unit of analysis in Bales's (1950) and other similar coding schemes is the utterance or sentence (or both) or thought unit. In analyzing relational control the unit of analysis is the exchange. Thus, it is possible to look for patterns of reciprocal influence of the interaction participants on one another and look for characteristic patterns such as one up, one down, and one across. These, in turn, relate to a continuum that goes from symmetry (maximum similarity) to complementarity (maximum difference).

One of the difficulties of trying to translate findings from one field or domain to another is that it is hard to know whether the results have practical significance. Both because the sample size is so small and the medical encounter is interactionally constrained in a way that contrasts with other more casual conversational or work contexts, it is difficult to know what the findings from von Friederichs-Fitzwater and Gilgun's study mean in practical terms. Perhaps, following Shaikh et al.'s logic about the context sensitivity of patient and physician roles, it would be useful to ask whether relational control patterns should be different in different phases of the encounter.

Like von Friederichs-Fitzwater and Gilgun's article, McNeilis's contribution to this issue focuses on the sequential relation between utterances and the extent to which findings about topic cohesion derived from studies of casual conversation can be applied fruitfully to the clinical encounter. Topic is a complex concept to apply in the medical encounter. There are points in the medical dialogue, the review of systems is a good example, where a series of unrelated closed ended, *yes* or *no* questions is typically and appropriately asked. Technically, each item on a review of systems checklist could be considered a change of topic. Alternatively, engaging in such behavior when eliciting the full spectrum of presenting concerns would interrupt the goal of understanding the narrative thread of the patient's illness experience. Because the same competency can have widely divergent acceptability and consequences depending on where and when it occurs, it is perhaps worth developing a taxonomy of competencies that are unique to the clinical context which may or may not have an analog in casual conversation. This would certainly help in interpreting the results reported here.

The article by Street and Millay targets patient participation in the medical encounter as desirable and analyzes nine of the taped encounters. Interestingly, these authors provide information about the ethnic composition of the sample and a gender breakdown of the physicians. No mention is made of the proportion of visits in which faculty preceptors were present nor their ethnicity or gender.

Street and Millay use both quantitative and qualitative methods to study patient participation using the exchange as their unit of analysis. As such, they are able to ask two key questions: (a) To what extent do patients in the sample ask questions, express concerns, and engage in assertive behavior? and (b) Are patients more likely to participate in these consultations when their physicians use partnership building and supportive talk? As the authors point out, these questions require different methodological approaches to answer. The quantitative analysis of the encounters showed a pattern which has been consistently found in the literature—baseline rates of patient participation are low, less than 7% of the total utterances for patients. Similarly physicians used partnership statements less than 2% of the time, but when they did it was reflected in more active participation. Use of the qualitative framework allowed the investigators to display the actual sequences in which this effect was seen. From a practical point of view this is helpful because it allows clinicians direct access to the performance patterns that increase and inhibit patient participation, an analytically and pedagogically sophisticated approach to the data and its analysis.

## CONCLUSIONS

What are the lessons learned from publishing this special Issue of *Health Communication*? The first lesson is that there is value in conducting the type of "thought experiment" that the contributors reflect. Not only does giving each contributor the same data to analyze reveal important theoretical and conceptual differences in approach, it also allows us to view where we are and where we may be going in the field of doctor–patient communication research. As someone who was trained in the "other" school of research (my first assignment as a graduate student with Harvey Sacks was to spend a year analyzing a 1 min fragment of a six-party conversation), I was disappointed not to see more of an attempt to achieve balance between the research types I identified in the beginning of this article. In fact, the benefits of combining approaches as Street and Millay have done in this issue are probably predictable. In a recent multiyear study that Wendy Levinson, Debra Roter, myself, and others (Levinson, Roter, Mullooly, Dull, & Frankel, 1997) conducted on the relation between physician–patient communication and medical malpractice, we consciously and actively sought to bring our two streams of work (quantitative and qualitative) together at the end of the project. When combined, the synthesis of both approaches had better predictive power than either one alone.

A second lesson is that it is important to recognize the value of developing standards for reporting research results. Given the diverse ways each of the investigators described the setting, criteria for inclusion and exclusion and the presence of third-party interactions when everyone was presumably describing the same data suggests that there is room for improvement. Because it is impossible, in principle, to reconstruct raw data from category codes unless a tape or transcript accompanies the analysis, it is worthwhile thinking about conventions for reporting that would minimize this source of variation.

A third lesson from this project is to recognize the incredible ingenuity and creativity that the investigators brought to their task. Whether it was using a general-purpose instrument to explore associations between communication behaviors and the task or phase of the encounter, or it was creating a method for targeting behaviors or sequences known to have a salutary effect on the care process and its outcomes, each investigator had developed a creative way to answer the question(s) raised. In my estimation the fact that the results varied across the six studies is an indication of the health of a relatively young field that is maturing rapidly. That having been said, it is important to stress again the importance of research question(s) determining method(s) and not the other way around (Frankel, 1999). A decontextualized debate about the inherent superiority of one method over another is about as useful as trying to pilot a nuclear submarine without navigation equipment or, on the other hand, equipping a canoe with 1,800 lb of sonar, radar, and GPS navigation equipment! It is impossible to get practical results unless you know what you are setting out to do and use the tools that are appropriate for the job.

Finally, a debt of gratitude goes to the editor of this special issue without whose foresight and hard work the project would never have taken place. It is a special honor and privilege for me to have the opportunity to share my thoughts about what is undeniably one of the most exciting frontiers of social science research. I agree with Albert von Szent-Gyorgi, who said in accepting the 1937 Nobel Prize in Physiology and Medicine, "Discovery consists of seeing what everybody has seen and thinking what nobody has thought."

## ACKNOWLEDGMENTS

I gratefully acknowledge Ronald Epstein, University of Rochester School of Medicine; Annsi Perakyla, University of Tempere, Finland; and Douglas Maynard, University of Wisconsin, for their helpful comments on this article.

## REFERENCES

Bales, R. F. (1950). *Interaction process analysis: A method for the study of small groups*. Reading, MA: Addison-Wesley.

Condon, W. S., & Ogston, W. D. (1967). A segmentation of behavior. *Journal of Psychiatric Research, 5*, 221–235.

Condon, W. S., & Ogston, W. D. (1971). Speech and body motions synchrony of the speaker and hearer. In D. L. Horton & J. J. Jenkins (Eds.), *Perceptions of language* (pp. 224–256). Westerville, OH: Merrill.

Frankel, R. M. (1999). Standards of qualitative research. In B. F. Crabtree & W. L. Miller (Eds.), *Doing qualitative research* (2nd ed., pp. 333–346). Thousand Oaks, CA: Sage.

Jordan, B., & Henderson, A. (1995). Interaction analysis: Foundations and practice. *The Journal of the Learning Sciences, 4,* 39–103.

Korsch, B. M., Gozzi, E. K., & Frances, V. (1968). Gaps in doctor–patient communication: 1. Doctor–patient interaction and patient satisfaction. *Pediatrics, 42,* 855–870.

Korsch, B. M., & Negrete, V. F. (1972). Doctor–patient communication. *Scientific American, 227,* 66–74.

Levinson, W. D., Roter, D. L., Mullooly, J., Dull, V., & Frankel, R. M. (1997). Physician–patient communication: The relationship with malpractice claims among primary care physicians and surgeons. *Journal of the American Medical Association, 277,* 553–559.

McQuown, N. E., Bateson, G., Birdwhistell, R. L., Brosen, H. W., & Hockett, C. F. (1971). *The natural history of an interview.* Chicago: University of Chicago Library, Microfilm Collection of Manuscripts in Cultural Anthropology.

Parsons, T. (1951). *The social system.* New York: Free Press.

Parsons, T., & Shills, E. (1952). *Toward a general theory of action.* Cambridge, MA: Harvard University Press.

Pittinger, R. E., Hockett, C. F., & Danehy, J. J. (1960). *The first five minutes.* Ithaca, NY: Martineau.

Roter, D. L. (1977). Patient participation in the patient–provider interaction: The effects of patient question asking on the quality of interaction, satisfaction and compliance. *Health Education Monographs, 5,* 281–315.

Roter, D., & Frankel, R. (1992). Quantitative and qualitative approaches to the evaluation of the medical dialogue. *Social Science & Medicine, 34,* 1097–1103.

Sheflen, A. (1971). *Communicational structure: Analysis of a psychotherapy transaction.* Bloomington: Indiana University Press.

Starfield, B., Steinwachs, D., Morris, I., Bause, G., Siebert, S., & Westin, C. (1979). Patient–doctor agreement about problems needing follow-up visit. *Journal of the American Medical Association, 242,* 344–346.

Starfield, B., Wray, C., Hess, K., Gross, R., Birk, P. S., & D'Lugoff, B. C. (1981). The influence of patient–practitioner agreement on outcome of care. *American Journal of Public Health, 71,* 127–131.

Stewart, M. (1995). Effective physician–patient communication and health outcomes: A review. *Canadian Medical Association Journal, 152,* 1423–1433.

Stewart, M., Brown, J. B., Boon, H., Galajda, J., Meredith, L., & Sangster, M. (1999). Evidence on patient–doctor communication. *Cancer Prevention Control, 3,* 25–30.

Stoeckle, J. D., & Billings, J. A. (1987). A history of history-taking: The medical interview. *Journal of General Internal Medicine, 2,* 119–127.

# BOOK REVIEWS

**Handbook of Communication and People With Disabilities: Research and Application.** Edited by Dawn O. Braithwaite and Teresa L. Thompson, Mahwah, NJ: Lawrence Erlbaum Associates, Inc., 2000, 555 pages, $125.00 (hardcover).

James Ferris
*Department of Communication Arts*
*University of Wisconsin, Madison*

The United States and the world are liberally endowed with people who have some sort of disability. Just how many people have a disability depends on who is doing the counting and how they decide whom to count. According to the United Nations Division for Social Policy and Development (2000), some 10% of the world's more than 6 billion people have some type of physical, mental, or sensory impairment. The U.S. Census Bureau (1997) must have been using a different yardstick when it estimated that one in five Americans has a disability—nearly 55 million people.

But however big the percentage, people with disabilities make up a considerable portion of the population, one that demands the attention of communication scholars. *Handbook of Communication and People With Disabilities,* the first attempt at a comprehensive collection of communication research on disability issues, shows that communication studies has not overlooked this important dimension of human experience.

Editors Teresa L. Thompson and Dawn O. Braithwaite are the leading scholars in communication studies who are investigating disability issues; each has been exploring such questions for at least 2 decades. Their goal with this book was to facilitate the efforts of future researchers and practitioners by gathering essays and literature reviews that focus on the central role of communication processes in the social construction of disability. The book's target audience extends beyond communication scholars to the wide range of social sciences, especially including psychology, social work, sociology, special education, anthropology, nursing, gerontology, and rehabilitation.

The handbook is ambitious, presenting mostly review-type chapters that draw from a wide variety of the perspectives and emphases that make up the communication discipline. This variety is a strength of the book, for it demonstrates the wide range of approaches that communication scholars are using to seek answers to questions about communication and disability. However, the book is enormous—it weighs in at more than 550 pages, with nearly 30 chapters by almost 50 authors. Fortunately, the handbook is relatively manageable. The chapters tend to be accessible, and the organization makes sense. The book is organized into five principal sections; the first four deal with interpersonal issues, organizational topics, cultural questions, and concerns related to media and technology. The fifth section explores communication questions as they pertain to a wide range of specific impairments.

The book's variety can be seen in the first section, which emphasizes interpersonal issues. The first chapter takes a dialectical perspective on the personal relationships of people with disabilities; the second examines the development and maintenance of romantic relationships between disabled and nondisabled partners, focusing particularly on the effects of socialization. Another chapter privileges narrative as it explores questions of identity and embodiment and provides insight into "trans-formation," the process of communicating in ways that transcend stereotypes. The section also includes a chapter that uses a resource theory perspective to examine the issue of help between disabled and nondisabled people, and one that takes a feminist phenomenological approach to explore how women with disabilities contest, accept, and transform societal meanings of disability.

And that's just the first section. The second section of the book focuses on disability-related communication issues in organizational contexts. Enhancing special education through the use of communication skills and strategies is the goal of one chapter, which suggests practices to promote effective communication among educators, students, parents, and professionals. Another chapter with an educational focus uses Dunkin and Biddle's (1974) model of teaching to explore communication concerns affecting students with disabilities on college campuses. Chapters also examine communication issues in the workplace. One looks at workplace communication issues around disability, especially in light of the requirements of the Americans with Disabilities Act (ADA); another calls attention to the 70% unemployment rate for people with disabilities and suggests communication strategies useful for disabled applicants in job interviews. The final chapter in this section urges modern organizations to meet the mandates of the ADA in spirit by moving beyond the introduction of adaptive devices such as ramps and modified computers to embrace a cultural ideology of pluralistic integration that will welcome the diversity represented by disabled people.

The next section of the book takes disability and culture as its focus. The first chapter reviews theoretical frameworks used to examine what the authors term *interability communication*—communication between disabled and nondisabled people—and then seeks to explain how psychosocial and cultural variables affect interability communication. That is followed by a chapter that uses identity-management theory to explain some of the ways that people with and without identified disabilities negotiate personal identities. The next chapter explores intercultural views of people with disabilities in Asia and Africa, then provides a more detailed look at disability in Japan, drawing on the experience of one of the authors, a native Japanese who has a disability. The section ends with a chapter that undertakes a rhetorical analysis of the goals of the disability movement, focusing particularly on deaf culture.

The fourth section of the handbook looks at issues related to communications media, including images of the disabled in televised, photographic, and print news; in film; and in advertising. Another chapter looks at the strengths and weaknesses of computer-mediated communication as an avenue of social support for disabled people.

The final major section of the book uses a variety of theoretical tools—ranging from uncertainty reduction theory to Bourdieu's (1991) concept of symbolic violence—to consider communication aspects of a range of impairments, including spinal cord injury, deafness, blindness, voicelessness, stuttering and other speaking difficulties, invisible disabilities, HIV/AIDS, and Alzheimer's disease.

In the concluding chapter, Braithwaite and Thompson sketch out future directions for communication and disability research. They suggest a number of important questions in the educational, organizational, interpersonal, and intercultural and cross-cultural realms that communication scholars have the tools to investigate fruitfully. They call for a new line of research into the communicative experiences of people with disabilities in health care contexts. Braithwaite and Thompson urge communication scholars to move beyond Goffman's (1986) stigma theory and embrace new theoretical perspectives, and they make a compelling call for careful and continued study of the mass media ranging from books to television to computers and emerging assistive technologies.

These are useful directions for researchers to take, but our discipline should be doing more. Recall that the proportion of disabled people in the United States is double that of the world. This large disparity suggests the extent to which disability is what Michael Bérubé (1998) called "the most labile and pliable of human categories," which makes disability "inevitably a matter of social debate and social construction" (pp. vii–viii). Disability is a socially constructed category similar to gender, race, ethnicity, and class. A discipline such as ours, rooted not only in the social sciences but also in the humanities, should be playing an important role in the growing critical discussion of disability. Scholars in rhetoric, performance studies, and critical and cultural studies, for example, should be examining the ways disability is created, embodied, manipulated, and performed by a society that presents as "normal" bodily ideals that can only be met by a very few people, and by them only for a limited time. Disability rights scholar Simi Linton (1998) argued that the absence of disability as a critical category of analysis weakens the knowledge base for the wide range of academic pursuits, for it robs us of all we can learn about the world—and how society has constructed the world—"from the vantage point of the atypical" (p. 5). Communication scholars have a great deal to contribute to the emerging interdisciplinary discussion that is disability studies, and as Braithwaite and Thompson argue, we should not limit our investigations to any one type of questions or any one set of tools. There is much to be done, and we must be about it.

*Handbook of Communication and People with Disabilities* is a landmark book, one of whose strengths is that it heeds Linton's (1998) call for disability research to prominently feature the voices of disabled people—one fourth of the authors in the book themselves have disabilities. It would be strengthened further, however, by another careful round of proofreading: The book's credibility is diminished somewhat by errors in scholars' names as well as in writing mechanics. This small concern aside, *Handbook of Communication and People with Disabilities* will be useful to scholars interested in communication questions around disability, for it provides a valuable sampling of many of the kinds of work that communication scholars are doing in this area. It will be of particular value as a textbook for the growing number of classes exploring communication and disability. More importantly, however, the book makes a significant contribution to disability studies because it highlights communication as a crucial factor in the social construction of disability. It is easy to assume when we talk about a social model of disability that communication is involved; this book shows some of the ways that disability is both communicated and communicative.

## REFERENCES

Bérubé, M. (1998). Foreword: Pressing the claim. In S. Linton, *Claiming disability: Knowledge and identity* (pp. vii–xi). New York: New York University Press.

Bureau of the Census. (1997). *Disabilities affect one-fifth of all Americans* (Census Brief 97–5).Washington, DC: Author. Retrieved January 23, 2001 from the World Wide Web: http://www.census.gov/hhes/www/disability.html

Bourdieu, P. (1991). *Language and symbolic power* (G. Raymond & M. Adamson, Trans.). Cambridge, MA: Harvard University Press.

Dunkin, M. J., & Biddle, B. J. (1974). *The study of teaching.* New York: Holt, Rinehart & Winston.

Goffman, E. (1986). *Stigma: Notes on the management of spoiled identity.* Englewood Cliffs, NJ: Prentice-Hall.

Linton, S. (1998). *Claiming disability: Knowledge and identity.* New York: New York University Press.

United Nations Division for Social Policy and Development. (2000). *Human rights and disabled persons.* Washington, DC: Author. Retrieved January 23, 2001 from the World Wide Web: http://www.un.org/Photos/disabled.htm

**Talking About Treatment.** Felicia D. Roberts, New York: Oxford University Press, 1999, $39.95 (hardcover).

Jeffrey D. Robinson
*Department of Speech Communicaion*
*Pennsylvania State University*

Roberts's book is an "attempt to fully describe and analyze the ways in which doctors and patients interact through language to create a forum in which recommendations for cancer treatment are given and received" (p. 105). Roberts's data, which are primarily a subsample of those collected by Siminoff (see Siminoff & Fetting, 1989, 1991; Siminoff, Fetting, & Abeloff, 1989), are 22 audiotaped consultations between nine different oncologists and women who have undergone surgery for breast cancer. These consultations center around discussions of, and recommendations for, adjuvant (i.e., additional, postoperative) treatments, such as chemotherapy, radiation, and hormonal therapy. Roberts's analyses are grounded in the theory and method of conversation analysis (for review, see Drew & Heritage, 1992; Heritage, 1984) and informed by a 6-week ethnography of an oncology center. All of the data are carefully transcribed using the conventions developed by Jefferson (1984).

The book contains six chapters. In chapter 1, "Research Concerns and Review of Literature," Roberts reviews research on quantitative and qualitative studies of medical interaction, cancer treatment recommendations, and the co-construction of medical power and expertise. In chapter 2, "Analytic Approach," Roberts justifies her use of conversation analysis and discusses her data, research procedures, and participants. In chapter 3, "Phased Organization of the Adjuvant Therapy Visit," Roberts analyzes the ordered phases, or activities, that regularly compose adjuvant consultations. Roberts lists these activities, describes their medical function(s), and analyzes "how the shape of the turns (who speaks and when) and the content (what is attended to as an appropriate contribution) construct these interactions as institutional service encounters which are legitimate occasions for giving and receiving recommendations" (p. 26). For example, Roberts analyzes how physicians and patients construct consultations as agenda based, service-encounter forums for giving advice. In chapter 4, "Discourse Identities: Establishing Participant Roles as Doctor and Patient," Roberts describes how physicians and patients construct "expertise," or lack thereof, as a social identity. Specifically, she analyzes the identity work involved in patients' requests for information and guidance, physicians' responses, and physicians' praise of patients' knowledge. Roberts works from the conversation-analytic premise that

> doctors are not expert service providers simply because they carry specialized knowledge in their heads; doctors are experts by virtue of (1) the expertise/knowledge they display or invoke in the encounter and (2) the conversational moves they initiate which establish them as gatekeepers to knowledge. (p. 51)

In chapter 5, "The Recommendation," Roberts analyzes how physicians and patients negotiate adjuvant treatment recommendations, including (a) the regular structure and content of, and argumentative strategies involved in, physicians' recommendations; (b) patients' responses, including how patients accept, question, or resist physicians' recommendations; and (c) physicians' subsequent moves, including how they advocate treatment and overcome patient resistance while simultaneously tempering patient optimism and diminishing patient pessimism. At the end of this chapter, Roberts deals very briefly with how physicians and patients close, or end, consultations. In Roberts's conclusion, she briefly summarizes her findings.

Roberts's book has both drawbacks and advantages. The first drawback is that the book is short—110 pages, excluding footnotes, references, and two appendixes. The three analytic chapters (chapters 3–5) comprise 79 pages. The length constrains what the book can accomplish. For instance, the review of the literature in chapter 1 is 15 pages, and constitutes more of a guided tour of references than a detailed review and critique of findings. For another example, Roberts's discussion of treatment recommendations in chapter 5 is 25 pages, and does not capture the entirety of the nuances of this interactionally large and complex activity. A second drawback is that the activity of physical examination was not audiorecorded and thus not analyzed, and researchers have demonstrated that other medical activities are coimplicated in physical examination (Heritage & Stivers, 1999; Stivers, 1998). A final drawback is that, in chapter 4, Roberts does not integrate her findings into those of certain discourse and conversation analysts who have examined asymmetries of physicians' and patients' knowledge (e.g., Drew, 1991; Linell, 1990; Linell & Luckmann, 1991).

Despite these drawbacks, Roberts's book represents the very first examination of adjuvant therapy consultations from an interactionist perspective. The book is insightful and illuminating and constructively contributes to existing discourse- and conversation-analytic research on physician–patient communication, both in terms of its analytic observations and the avenues they open for future research. In addition to single sequences of talk, Roberts addresses larger scale structures of medical interaction. In some cases, such as in chapter 4, Roberts begins to analyze phenomena that have largely not been addressed by previous researchers, such as physicians' praise of patients. Furthermore, Roberts provides a detailed analysis of treatment recommendations in a context of medicine other than primary care. Her findings begin to expose cross-contextual similarities and differences regarding treatment and thus heuristically contribute to an understanding of treatment as a general medical activity that gets interactionally tailored to particular medical contexts and goals.

Roberts's book certainly belongs in the personal libraries of all researchers interested in the processual details of physician–patient communication, especially those interested in how participants construct and manage interactional control and social identities. Although Roberts does not address how her communication (i.e., process) variables (e.g., patients' questions, physicians' praise, etc.) relate to input or demographic variables or medical outcomes, her findings certainly shed light on the types of process variables that are relevant in adjuvant treatment consultations and how these variables might be operationalized for the purposes of coding. In sum, Roberts's book should be of interest to a wide range of researchers interested in physician–patient communication.

## REFERENCES

Drew, P. (1991). Asymmetries of knowledge in conversational interactions. In I. Markova & K. Foppa (Eds.), *Asymmetries in dialogue* (pp. 29–48). Savage, MA: Barnes & Noble.

Drew, P., & Heritage, J. (1992). Analyzing talk at work: An introduction. In P. Drew & J. Heritage (Eds.), *Talk at work: Interaction in institutional settings* (pp. 3–65). Cambridge, England: Cambridge University Press.

Heritage, J. (1984). *Garfinkel and ethnomethodology.* Cambridge, England: Polity.

Heritage, J., & Stivers, T. (1999). Online commentary in acute medical visits: A method of shaping patient expectations. *Social Science & Medicine, 49,* 1501–1517.

Jefferson, G. (1984). Transcription notation. In J. M. Atkinson & J. Heritage (Eds.), *Structures of social action: Studies in conversation analysis* (pp. ix–xvi). Cambridge, England: Cambridge University Press.

Linell, P. (1990). The power of dialogue dynamics. In I. Markova & K. Foppa (Eds.), *The dynamics of dialogue* (pp. 147–177). Hemel Hempstead, England: Harvester Wheatsheaf.

Linell, P., & Luckmann, T. (1991). Asymmetries in dialogue: Some conceptual preliminaries. In I. Markova & K. Foppa (Eds.). *Asymmetries in dialogue* (pp. 1–31). Savage, MA: Barnes & Noble.

Siminoff, L. A., & Fetting, J. H. (1989). Effects of outcome framing on treatment decisions in the real world. *Medical Decision Making, 9,* 262–271.

Siminoff, L. A., & Fetting, J. H. (1991). Factors affecting treatment decisions for a life threatening illness: The case of medical treatment of breast cancer. *Social Science and Medicine, 32,* 813–818.

Siminoff, L. A., Fetting, J. H., & Abeloff, M. D. (1989). Doctor–patient communication about breast cancer adjuvant therapy. *Journal of Clinical Oncology, 7,* 1192–1200.

Stivers, T. (1998). Prediagnostic commentary in veterinarian–client interaction. *Research on Language and Social Interaction, 31,* 241–277.

Milton Keynes UK
Ingram Content Group UK Ltd.
UKHW022109141024
449569UK00031B/1844